D1743867

Speech Disorders in Adults

Recent Advances

Editor in chief, Speech, Language, and Hearing Disorders Series
William H. Perkins, PhD

Speech Disorders in Adults

Recent Advances

edited by

Janis M. Costello, PhD

Speech and Hearing Center

University of California, Santa Barbara

NFER-NELSON

First published in Great Britain 1985 by The NFER-NELSON Publishing Company Ltd., Darville House, 2 Oxford Road East, Windsor, Berkshire SL4 1DF.

First published in the USA 1985 by College Hill Press Inc
4284 41st Street
San Diego, California 92105
© 1985 by College-Hill Press Inc.

Code 8867 02 1

ISBN 0 7005 1018 4

Library of Congress Cataloging in Publication Data

Costello, Janis M.
  Speech disorders in adults

    Includes bibliographies and indexes

    1. Speech, Disorders of.   2. Voice disorders.
    3. Stuttering.   I. Costello, Janis M.
[DNLM: 1. Speech Disorders.   2. Voice Disorders.   WM 475 57424]
RC423.S63828   1985   616.85′5   84–29199

Printed in the United States of America.

PUBLISHER'S NOTE

These volumes were developed under the supervision of a group of leading scientists charged with the responsibility of assessing the most critical book needs of the speech-language-hearing profession. In consultation with William H. Perkins and Raymond G. Daniloff, serving as editors in chief of the ensuing volumes on speech, language, and hearing disorders (Perkins) and speech, language, and hearing science (Daniloff), the publisher planned a series of nine mutually independent texts covering the entirety of state-of-the-art knowledge in these disciplines, with contributions by respected, productive, and current scholars known for their expertise as specialists in key areas.

Each contribution has been stringently refereed for content, pedagogy, and practical value for students and practitioners by the individual volume editors, Charles Berlin, Janis Costello, Raymond Daniloff, Audrey Holland, James Jerger, Rita Naremore, and their designated reviewers, in close consultation throughout with the editors in chief and the publisher. Users are thus assured that their needs for accurate, timely information, reflecting the highest standards of scholarship and professionalism, have been faithfully met.

On behalf of the speech-language-hearing profession, its researchers, teachers, practitioners, and students, present and future, the publisher thanks the more than 100 authors and editors who have given generously of their time and knowledge to produce this magnificient contribution to the literature.

Speech Disorders in Adults, edited by Janis M. Costello, is one of nine state-of-the-art volumes comprising the College-Hill Press series covering the current body of knowledge in speech, language, and hearing.

Volume Titles:	Editors:
Speech Disorders in Children	Janis M. Costello
Speech Disorders in Adults	Janis M. Costello
Speech Science	Raymond Daniloff
Language Disorders in Children	Audrey Holland
Language Disorders in Adults	Audrey Holland
Language Science	Rita Naremore
Pediatric Audiology	James Jerger
Hearing Disorders in Adults	James Jerger
Hearing Science	Charles Berlin

Editor in Chief, Speech, Language, and Hearing Disorders Series:	William H. Perkins
Editor in Chief, Speech, Language, and Hearing Science Series:	Raymond G. Daniloff

CONTENTS

CONTRIBUTORS

James Abbs, Ph.D.
Waisman Center
Speech Motor Control
  Laboratories
University of Wisconsin
Madison, WI

Janis M. Costello, Ph.D.
Speech and Hearing Center
University of California, Santa
  Barbara
Santa Barbara, CA

M. N. Hegde, Ph.D.
Department of Communicative
  Disorders
California State University at
  Fresno
Fresno, CA

Roger Ingham, Ph.D.
Speech and Hearing Center
University of California, Santa
  Barbara
Santa Barbara, CA

Thomas S. Johnson, Ph.D.
Department of Communication
  Disorders
Utah State University
Logan, UT

Jeri A. Logemann, Ph.D.
Northwestern University
Evanston, IL

William H. Perkins, Ph.D.
Center for the Study of
  Communication Disorders
University of Southern California
Los Angeles, CA

John C. Rosenbek, Ph.D.
Speech Pathology and Audiology
Veterans Administration Hospital
Madison, WI

Bernd Weinberg, Ph.D.
Department of Audiology and
  Speech Sciences
Purdue University
West Lafayette, IN

Walter A. Wolfram, Ph.D.
University of the District of
  Columbia
Washington, DC

FOREWORD

From 1977 to 1982, while editing the *Journal of Speech and Hearing Disorders,* I became increasingly aware of the rate at which information about communication disorders was expanding. Not only was it an information explosion, it was a conceptual explosion as well, particularly in the area of children's language. We are departing rapidly from a relatively insular profession in which clinical practice has been based largely on what we could learn from our own experience. What we are moving toward is a theory-based profession in which we are open to broad-ranging conceptions, most notably from linguistics, medicine, and psychology.

It was against this background that *Recent Advances: Speech, Language, and Hearing Pathology* was spawned. In accepting the responsibility of being Editor in Chief, I saw several opportunities. Above all, it offered a vehicle by which the profession could remain current. Some areas have moved so rapidly that they bear little resemblance to what they were even a decade ago. Not only has information proliferated, but so have the journals and texts in which it has been preserved. Here, then, in *Recent Advances,* was an opportunity to organize a coherent and comprehensive account of the current state of affairs in all clinical aspects of speech, language, and hearing.

A price paid for advancement of knowledge is not only inability to consume the increasing glut, but even to comprehend it. One must almost be a specialist to understand what other specialists are talking about. To chronicle the state of the art across all areas of communication disorders, and still make responsible statements, would require the best minds available in each area. To know who these experts are, and to obtain their participation, would require scholars of such stature as to attract them. Hence, my most important responsibility in this project was the selection of volume editors. I take great pride that Janis Costello, Audrey Holland, and James Jerger agreed to participate.

With their respective editorships established, my remaining responsibility was to consult with them in determining the chapters needed to report the state of the art in their areas, and in selecting authors most qualified to prepare the chapters. We sought authors who not only are established scholars, but who also write with clarity. We were as concerned that anyone in the profession be able to read and understand what is going on in any area as we were with assembling the best information available.

Aside from nudging the project along occasionally and final editing, I can claim little credit for the sterling quality of these tests. That credit belongs to the editors.

William H. Perkins
Editor in chief

PREFACE

As was true of our efforts in the earlier volume, *Speech Disorders in Children: Recent Advances,* this volume on the assessment and management of speech disorders among adult populations is a compilation, authored by the best qualified researcher-clinicians, of recent research and critical thought regarding articulatory disorders, second language (phonology) acquisition, voice disorders, and stuttering. These chapters illustrate in an eloquent fashion the rapid increase in knowledge that is occurring, seemingly daily, in each of these areas, and they provide a framework for weaving this new information into the fabric of our current knowledge. For those of us who find ourselves increasingly unable to keep up with new developments, these authors give us a chance to catch up, at least for a time.

This volume is divided into separate sections on recent advances in adult articulation and phonology, voice disorders, and stuttering. Each section is introduced by a chapter that provides an overview of the major developments in the area in order to set the scene for the description of recent advances in specific areas. Each of the chapters on recent advances concentrates on major work carried out within the last few years, although the classic studies that often served as the impetus for work being produced now are generally described as well.

It is a healthy sign for our discipline and profession that a series of *Recent Advances* volumes is needed. Let's hope that our health continues to blossom and that this injection of new knowledge will serve to stimulate still more in the future, thus providing a sturdy base for continued growth and enhanced clinical services to speech disordered adults.

Janis M. Costello
Editor

Part I
Articulation and
Phonology

Chapter 1

Assessment and Treatment of Articulatory Disorders in Adults: State of the Art

Jeri A. Logemann

Adult articulation disorders are typically neurologically or anatomically based. They result from damage to neurologic control of the vocal tract (as in stroke, head trauma, and neurologic disease), to the muscles that produce changes in vocal tract shape for speech (as in muscular dystrophy), or to the structures of the vocal tract themselves (as in surgical or traumatic ablation) (Canter, 1964; Darley, Aronson, and Brown, 1968; Joanette and Dudley, 1980; Nakano, Zubick, and Tyler, 1973; Summers, 1974). In the main, these disorders are acquired well after the adult has attained a normal receptive and expressive phonologic system.

Figure 1-1 presents a schema for an optimal knowledge base in the area of acquired adult articulation disorders, against which currently available data can be compared. As a basis for all diagnosis and treatment planning, the exact nature of each disorder should be understood, beginning with the anatomic and physiologic changes created in the structures of the vocal tract and their movement patterns during speech. This information should be available in order to interpret the acoustic and perceptual characteristics of the disorder, because it has become apparent that more than one vocal tract gesture can produce the same acoustic or perceptual result.

In addition to a basic understanding of the nature of each disorder, its natural course must be documented in order for clinicians to diagnose and treat it optimally. Many of these acquired disorders result from trauma (e.g., stroke, head trauma, injury) or surgery, from which some recovery can be anticipated. Others are related to progressive neurologic disease (e.g.,

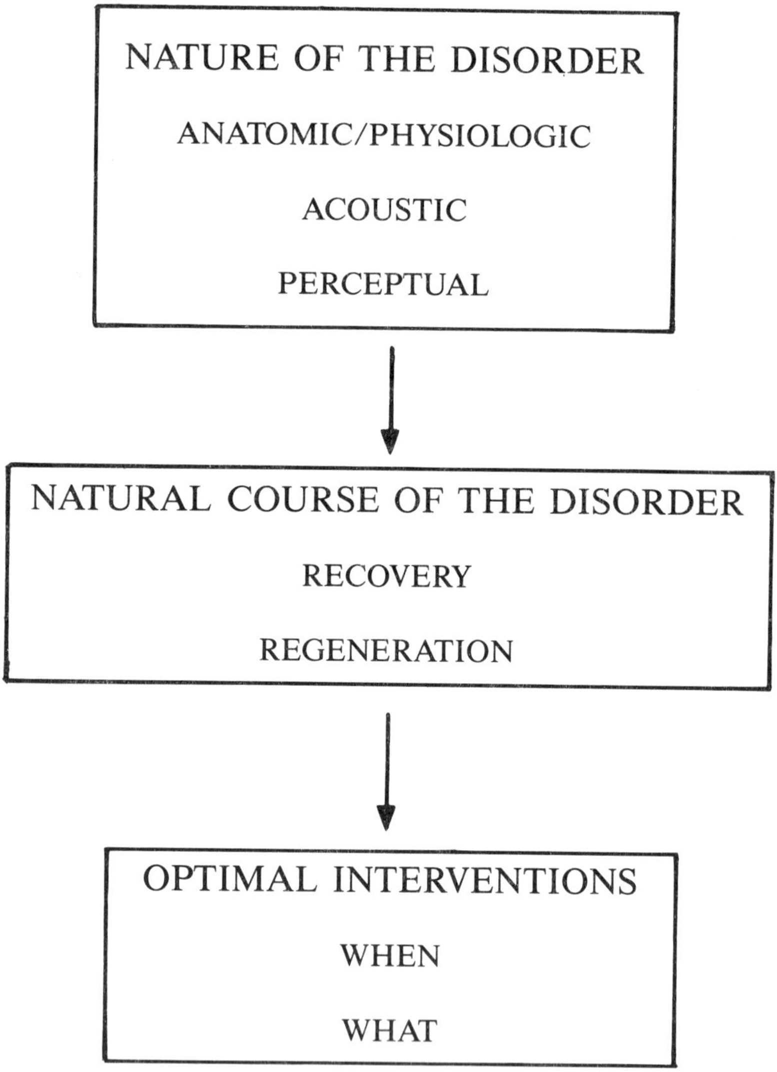

NATURE OF THE DISORDER

ANATOMIC/PHYSIOLOGIC

ACOUSTIC

PERCEPTUAL

↓

NATURAL COURSE OF THE DISORDER

RECOVERY

REGENERATION

↓

OPTIMAL INTERVENTIONS

WHEN

WHAT

Figure 1-1. An optimal data base for the understanding, diagnosis, and management of acquired adult articulation disorders.

amyotrophic lateral sclerosis, multiple sclerosis, Parkinson's disease) which will cause increasing decrement in function. Thus, data on the nature of the disorder must be collected longitudinally to determine the anatomic and physiologic changes that can be anticipated with recovery or with degeneration.

Finally, with detailed information on the nature of the disorder and its natural course, clinical investigators can design and evaluate optimal treatment strategies and can determine the best time for their introduction in the recovery or degenerative process.

DISORDERS OF NEUROLOGIC ORIGIN

Neurogenic disorders affecting the articulation patterns of adults are often the most complex because they can affect the function of the entire vocal tract—including the oral cavity, pharynx, larynx, and respiratory system—rather than the movement of a single articulator. These acquired neurogenic articulation disorders in adults must be considered, then, in the broadest sense, as movement disorders of the entire speech production mechanism (Kent and Netsell, 1975; Netsell, Daniel, and Celesia, 1975).

In the case of *apraxia*, the disorder results from cortical damage to the areas controlling motor programming, but is manifested as a disturbance in the normal movement patterns of the vocal tract to produce phonemic sequences (La Pointe and Johns, 1975; Trost and Canter, 1974; Wertz, La Pointe, and Rosenbek, 1984).

In the *dysarthrias*, the neuromotor behaviors involved in reaching a sequence of articulatory targets in connected speech are no longer executed normally. The locations and nature of the damage to the controls of these behaviors are not entirely understood, nor is the way in which damage to the neuromotor system translates into muscle function for vocal tract movement during speech production.

Evaluation of Articulatory Disorders of Neurologic Origin

Many of the early studies of the nature of apraxia and dysarthrias required trained listeners to analyze the error articulations and describe the voice disorders produced by each patient (Berry, Darley, Aronson, and Goldstein, 1973; Brown, Darley, and Aronson, 1970; Burns and Canter,

1977; Critchley, 1981; Darley, Aronson, and Brown, 1968, 1969, 1975; Farmakides and Boone, 1970; Linebaugh, 1979; Logemann, Boshes, Blonsky, and Fisher, 1977; Logemann and Fisher, 1981; Mawdesley, 1973; Peacher, 1947, 1950). The goal of these attempts was to construct a list of descriptive terms to be used diagnostically to distinguish apraxia and the various dysarthrias from each other and from other acquired articulation problems. Most of these investigators were also seeking to define the nature of the disorders as they affected some or all of the vocal tract. In reality, the descriptive terminology was often imprecise and usually overlapped across the various disorders, making discrimination among them difficult.

In examining the nature of apraxia, many investigators have concentrated on phonetic analyses of the patients' productions (Johns and Darley, 1970; La Pointe and Johns, 1975; Trost and Canter, 1974). Other investigators have quantified the changes in vocal tract control in apraxia and the dysarthrias through assessment of specific acoustic parameters (Blumstein, Cooper, Goodglass, Statlender, and Gottleib, 1980; Kent and Netsell, 1975; Kent, Netsell, and Abbs, 1979; Lehiste, 1968; Ludlow and Bassich, 1982). For example, Kent and colleagues (1979) conducted an acoustic study of the dysarthria associated with cerebellar disease. They examined the speech of five persons with ataxic dysarthria, including an acoustic analysis of consonant-vowel-consonant (CVC) words, words of varying syllabic structure, simple sentences, the Rainbow passage, and conversation. The most consistent and marked abnormalities observed in the spectrograms were alterations of normal timing patterns with prolongation of several speech segments and a tendency toward equalizing the duration of the syllables. The formant structure of vowels in the CVC words was judged to be essentially normal except for the transitions into and away from the segments. The more severe the dysarthria, the larger the number of segments lengthened and the greater the degree of lengthening. This strengthens the concept of cerebellar control of rate of movement by the maintenance of normal targeting behavior. In discussing the results of their work, the authors suggest that the effects of speech therapy, medication, surgery, or other intervention strategies for patients may be more accurately and simply measured through these acoustic techniques.

Some investigators have attempted to relate acoustic measures to the perceptual judgments of listeners. In 1982, Ludlow and Bassich conducted a study of two types of dysarthric patients: parkinsonian patients and those with Shy-Drager syndrome. The purpose of this study was to determine whether acoustic measures of the speech of dysarthric patients differentiated their impairment from normal as well as perceptual ratings. The results indicated that, in fact, the two types of dysarthria could be distinguished from normal by both the acoustic measures and the perceptual ratings of speech. However, to distinguish the two types of dysarthria from each other, a composite score of several measures was necessary, indicating that a pattern of impairment rather than the degree of impairment is important in characterizing the patient's speech disorder.

Currently, several new, relatively noninvasive instrumentation techniques are being applied to the physiologic study of the nature of vocal tract movement patterns in neurologically impaired patients (Hirose, Kiritani, Ushijima, and Sawashima, 1978; Itoh, Sasanuma, Hirose, Yoshioka, and Ushijima, 1980; Kiritani, Ito, and Fujimura, 1975; Sonies, 1982; Sonies, Shauker, and Stowe, 1982). X-ray microbeam study of pellet movement during speech permits assessment of movement patterns of preselected points in the vocal tract as well as simultaneous acoustic and other physiologic measures. Ultrasound techniques may add to our understanding of the function of specific tongue musculature during speech production. Studies utilizing these procedures will add to our knowledge of speech movement patterns in apraxic and dysarthric patients—information previously collected through more traditional methods (Blonsky, Logemann, Boshes, and Fisher, 1975; Canter, 1963, 1965a, 1965b; Hardy, 1965; Hirose, 1971; Iwata, von Leden, and Williams, 1972; Kent and Netsell, 1975; Leanderson, Meyerson, and Persson, 1972; Meyerson, 1973).

Other noninvasive techniques for more accurate *clinical* assessment of vocal tract physiology are being developed and refined for application to the study of adults with acquired articulation disorders. For example, Netsell and Hixon (1978) have developed a noninvasive method for clinically estimating subglottal air pressure. This technique permits estimation of the driving pressure to the larynx and upper airway delivered by the respiratory system during speech production. This kind of examination can help the clinician to determine whether respiratory drive is sufficient to produce good laryngeal tone in the neurologically impaired patient, and thus can determine whether reduced respiratory control is a significant aspect of the patient's speech disorder. Barlow and Abbs (1983) have developed force transducers for the evaluation of labial, lingual, and mandibular motion impairments. This instrument will permit assessment of the motor control integrity of each motor subsystem independently. As other physiologic assessment procedures are simplified for clinical use, a routine battery of tests may be developed for use in diagnosis and management of neurologically impaired patients with speech motor control disturbances. Such a battery is sorely needed.

From this brief review of research on the nature of apraxia and the dysarthrias, it is evident that our current data base contains a large number of perceptual studies of the speech output of patients with these disorders, a moderate number of acoustic analyses of their speech productions, fewer studies of the physiologic nature of these movement disorders for speech, and very few investigations that assess and relate all three aspects of vocal tract dysfunctions.

Very few of the studies of dysarthria and apraxia have examined patients longitudinally to assess predictability of recovery or deterioration in neuromotor control of the vocal tract (Dworkin and Hartman, 1979; Logemann, Boshes, and Fisher, 1973; Mackay, 1963; Rigrodsky and Morrison, 1970). Nor have many investigations systematically assessed the effects of medication on movement disorders of the vocal tract (Birkmayer and Hornykiewicz, 1961). Often, any systematic changes with time have been obliterated by heterogeneous populations of patients, differing either in diagnosis, stage of disease, current medications, or time after onset.

When an adult is initially seen by a speech pathologist for evaluation and treatment of an articulation disorder, the first issue to be addressed is differential diagnosis. Since articulatory disorders in adults can signal the onset of degenerative neurologic diseases of various types, the clinician should be able to compare results of neuromotor testing of the patient's vocal tract control with an information base on typical patterns of change over time on selected measures in patients with specific neurologic diseases. Unfortunately, such a data base is not available. Very few studies have followed up patients longitudinally or have classified patients according to the stage of disease or the time after onset of symptoms. Dworkin and Hartman (1979) followed up a patient with amyotrophic lateral sclerosis to assess the progression in speech deterioration and swallowing. They found a relatively rapid deterioration, including reduction in tongue strength and rate of tongue movement, rate and strength of velopharyngeal function, and laryngeal disturbance.

Logemann and Fisher (1981) and Logemann, Fisher, Boshes, and Blonsky (1978) examined parkinsonian patients at various stages of the disease and found a systematic increase in the phonemes (and vocal tract structures) involved as the disease stage worsened. Unfortunately, few of these studies have included acoustic, physiologic, and perceptual analyses, so that firm conclusions regarding changes in vocal tract movement patterns over time could not be made.

Intervention Strategies for Articulatory Disorders of Neurologic Origin

Development of effective intervention strategies suffers from the lack of basic information on the nature of the disorders and their progression over time (recovery or deterioration). However, in the past ten years, clear trends in management have emerged. First, some clinical investigators are using physiologic and acoustic measures to analyze the patient's movement disorder(s) and to identify those components contributing most significantly to overall intelligibility (e.g., respiratory control, velopharyngeal incompetence) and are then focusing intervention strategies on the parameters so identified (Netsell and Daniel, 1979). These investigators and others are then applying the physiologic or acoustic measures to the evaluation of the interventions as they are implemented.

Second, several techniques to enhance the patient's feedback or awareness of specific vocal tract movements are being evaluated (Daniel and Guitar, 1978; Hanson and Metter, 1980; Netsell and Cleeland, 1973; Rubow, Rosenbek, Collins, and Celesia, 1984). In several reports, lip function has been improved with electromyographic (EMG) biofeedback. In a study by Hand, Burns, and Ireland (1979), a patient with lip hypertonia and retraction was treated with EMG biofeedback in order to demonstrate a reduction in postural lip hypertonicity and to demonstrate that reduction during a number of complex speech activities. The patient's hypertonicity decreased over six biofeedback sessions. It was hypothesized that the hypertonicity decreased because of reduced anisometric contraction, a reduction of isometric contraction, or a relearning of agonist and antagonist muscle balance. Several other authors have demonstrated ability to reduce lip hypertonia in parkinson patients by use of EMG biofeedback (Netsell and Cleeland, 1973).

Third, prosthetic techniques are being increasingly used as intervention strategies in these patients, including bite block prostheses (Lybolt, Netsell, and Farrage, 1982), palatal lift prostheses (Netsell and Daniel, 1979; Schweiger, Netsell, and Sommerfield, 1970), and palatal reshaping prostheses. In each case, the prosthesis is designed to increase functional capacity of particular articulators within the vocal tract. For example, the palatal lift prosthesis elevates the palate to facilitate velopharyngeal closure. A palatal augmentation reshaping prosthesis lowers the palate to meet the tongue that does not elevate sufficiently.

ADULTS WITH SPEECH DISORDERS RESULTING FROM ABLATION OF VOCAL TRACT STRUCTURES

As in adults with neurologically based articulation disorders, the earliest studies, and the greatest number of investigations on the nature of speech changes in patients after ablation of vocal tract structures, have examined perceptual and acoustic differences.

Peacher (1947), Herberman (1958), and Brodnitz (1960) described the postoperative speech patterns of their glossectomized subjects by noting the particular phonemes that proved to be the most difficult to produce. Skelly and associates (Donaldson, Skelly, and Paletta, 1968; Skelly, Donaldson, Fust, and Townsend, 1972; Skelly, Donaldson, and Fust, 1973; Skelly, Spector, Donaldson, Brodeur, and Paletta, 1971) have reported some information concerning the intelligibility scores of their glossectomized patients. In an unpublished paper presented at the 1972 American Speech and Hearing Association convention, Seilo, La Riviere, and Dimmick (1972) reported intelligibility scores of a glossectomy patient as determined by listener response to the reading of two word lists from the Rhyme Test (Fairbanks, 1958) and to the production of five vowels and three diphthongs in an [h] CVC context. In addition, they provided a confusion matrix for initial consonants as assessed by three "experienced listeners."

In any attempt to assess the relationship between structure and speech function in the patient after ablation of vocal tract structures, it is not sufficient to merely specify acoustic and perceptual changes or residual tissue structure and mobility. It is necessary to define accurately and objectively the characteristics of vocal tract movement during speech. Radiographic studies of articulatory gestures completed by Logemann and Bytell (1979), Logemann, Fisher, and Bytell (1982), Georgian, Logemann, and Fisher (1982), and Lazarus and Logemann (1982), have defined specific changes in vocal tract movement patterns after ablative surgery. The relationship between listener preception, acoustic features, and these productions has also been explored (Georgian, Logemann, and Fisher, 1982; Lazarus and Logemann, 1982).

Several investigators have found there is a minimal inter- and intrasubject variability in speech and swallowing measures when patients are carefully categorized according to the extent and nature of their ablative and reconstructive procedures. When functional changes in speech articulation patterns were compared across groups by Logemann and Bytell (1978), Logemann, Fisher, and Bytell (1977), and McConnell (1982), it was clear that each group of patients categorized by data on their resection-reconstruction procedures had a distinct profile of functioning that was different in the detailed characteristics of speech articulation and in the resultant acoustic and perceptual parameters. When Logemann and Bytell (1978) and McConnell (1982) categorized surgically treated oral cancer patients by extent of resection and nature of reconstruction, it became apparent that the severity of changes in speech articulation patterns after surgery related to the extent of the lingual resection and the nature of the reconstruction, *nature of the reconstruction* being the most important predictor of function in patients with less that one half of the tongue included in the resection, and *extent of resection* the most important predictor of function when more than 50 per cent of the tongue was resected. This research has clarified the role of surgical reconstruction as the foremost rehabilitation strategy. A number of surgeons are attempting improvements in oral reconstruction. Unfortunately, their results often are not examined in a careful, detailed, and systematic way in terms of their effect on speech movement patterns, acoustic characteristics, or listener perceptions.

Only a small amount of physiologic, acoustic, and perceptual data on recovery of more normal speech articulations by postoperative oral cancer patients, with and without therapeutic interventions, is available (Brodnitz, 1960; Duguay, 1964; Georgian, Logemann, and Fisher, 1982; Herberman, 1958; Seilo et al., 1972; Lazarus and Logemann, 1982). Although it is clear that the same acoustic and perceptual result can be created by more than one vocal tract gesture, our knowledge of which specific articulatory strategies produce the same perceptual judgments by the listener is minimal and is insufficient to apply in teaching patients optimal compensatory articulation strategies. The most frequent intervention described in the clinical literature involves development of intraoral prostheses to compensate for the loss of range of movement in vocal tract structures (Cantor, Curtis, Shipp, Beumer, and Vogel, 1969; Lehman, Hulicka, and Mehringer, 1966; Leonard and Gillis, 1982; Logemann, Sisson, and Wheeler, 1980; Moore, 1972; Wheeler, Logemann, and Rosen, 1980). Two basic approaches have been utilized in prosthetic rehabilitation of the oral cancer patient: maxillary prostheses designed to lower and reshape the palatal vault and thus facilitate contact of the residual tongue to the palate (Cantor et al. 1969; Logemann et al., 1980; Wheeler et al., 1980), and mandibular prosthetics with some attempt made to create a "prosthetic tongue" to improve intelligibility after essentially total glossectomy (Leonard and Gillis, 1982; Moore, 1972).

The timing of introduction of these prosthetic devices is currently open to question, with some investigators advocating early implementation with redesign as function recovers (Logemann et al., 1980), and other clinicians suggesting introduction of prostheses once the patient's function has reached a plateau, some time after the ablative incident (Drane, 1973).

AUGMENTATIVE COMMUNICATION STRATEGIES

Over the past ten years, speech-language pathologists have increasingly recognized the need to offer communication aids to patients whose speech is unintelligible (Coleman, Cook, and Meyers, 1980; Copeland, 1974, Skelly, Schinsky, Smith, and Fust, 1974; Vanderheiden and Grilley, 1976). Much of the attention in the area of alternative communication has focused on development and application of communication aids and systems for multiply handicapped children whose cognitive and language skills are just developing or are impaired (McDonald and Schultz, 1973; Montgomery, 1983; Shane and Bashir, 1980; Vanderheiden, Kelso, Holt, and Raitzer, 1977). In contrast to the special needs of these multiply handicapped children, most of the adults with acquired articulation disorders have normal receptive and expressive language, can solve problems, and can see relationships. They merely lack adequate intelligible speech to meet all of their communication needs (Beukelman and Yorkston, 1977; Silverman, 1983).

Initially, the alternative communication systems used by these speech impaired adults were manual (signing, gesturing, writing) or varieties of communication boards (Calculator and Dollaghan, 1982; Skelly et al., 1974). More recently, electronic devices, including computer systems producing digitized speech output, have been developed (Linebaugh, Baird, and Baird, 1983). Several authors have described the devices currently available, and many hospitals have now organized laboratories or centers for alternative communication as resources to speech-language and hearing professionals and patients in their communities (Linebaugh, Baird, Baird and Armour, 1983; Vanderheiden and Grilley, 1976). These centers purchase and maintain samples of a wide variety of alternative communication systems, which patients can see and use on a trial basis. Since many of these devices are quite expensive and cannot be purchased by each hospital or clinic for trial use by patients, the concept of the alternative communication center as a community resource is an excellent one. Many of the centers offer consultation and evaluation services to speech-language pathologists and their patients in the community regarding selection of the best system for a particular patient.

Several major problems currently face clinicians in selection of an instrument with and for a patient: maintaining a working knowledge of the advantages and disadvantages of the ever-increasing number and types of prosthetic devices available, and identifying the relevant criteria for selection of a device with and for a patient. The first problem is partially solved by the alternative communication centers just described. Unfortunately, however, very few of the available alternative communication systems have been evaluated in controlled studies of their utility, listener acceptance, patient acceptance, and effect on recovering oral communication with various types of patients.

Criteria for selection of a particular instrument by and for a particular patient have not been uniformly agreed upon. Several models for decision making have been offered in the literature (Coleman et al., 1980; Owens and House, 1984; Shane and Bashir, 1980). Each author has attempted to construct a type of decision tree or logic diagram to parallel the questions the clinician should answer or ask about the patient's capabilities in the process of selecting an instrument for a particular patient. Few studies have described the typical length of use of various systems or problems encountered, including the need to change systems as any of the patient's neuromotor, linguistic, or cognitive abilities or communication needs change.

The counseling process for patients and families when the speech-language pathologist believes alternative methods of communications are needed has received little attention. Yet, this recommendation by the clinician may arouse strong feelings of failure, inadequacy, and lack of acceptance in the patient and family if the information on the patient's need for such aids is not carefully introduced and reinforced. In some cases, the patient and family may believe the clinician is abandoning them or giving up on the goal of recovering or maintaining intelligible speech. In other cases, the move to an alternative communication system may signal one more loss in function in the face of progressive neurologic disease or malignancy. The role of the speech-language pathologist in counseling, reinforcement, and support, in conjunction with other professionals, deserves greater attention.

Though the number and electronic complexity of available electronic augmentation communication systems are increasing, several limitations still exist. First, the devices that produce digitized speech are not always easily intelligible to naive listeners, and often sound mechanical. Second, the size of many devices makes them less mobile than is desired by many patients, especially those who are ambulatory. Third, the cost of many of the better instruments makes them unavailable to many patients, particularly many older persons with limited resources that have already been strained by long illness, hospitalizations, and the like.

Thus, many advances have been made in the use of alternative communication systems by adults with acquired articulation disorders. However, much additional research and development are needed before optimal devices and procedures for their selection and introduction to patients are available.

SUMMARY

Many of the discrepancies between the ideal information base illustrated in Figure 1-1, and the current state of the art in adult articulation disorders as described here, relate to the difficulties in implementation of the research needed to expand our information base.

First, physiologic techniques that permit easy, relatively noninvasive study of movement patterns of vocal tract structures during speech in a large number of subjects are just beginning to be developed and used to study disorder groups (Hirose et al., 1978; Kiritani et al., 1975; Sonies, 1982). Simultaneous studies of movement patterns, air flows and pressures, EMG in select muscle groups, and other physiologic and acoustic measures are needed but require complex instrumentation not widely available. In place of these physiologic studies, many investigators have substituted acoustic and perceptual evaluations of various types of adult patients with acquired articulation disorders, recognizing the limitations of their results in extrapolating the underlying anatomic or physiologic nature of the disorder. To date, the majority of physiologic studies that have been completed examined only a small number of patients. How and where these individual patients fit into the continuum of recovery or degeneration of the disease entity they represent is often difficult for the reader to know.

Few studies have followed up specific homogeneous patient groups longitudinally to define patterns of recovery or degeneration. Availability of large homogeneous groups of patients early in their diagnosis is a problem for many investigators not located in major medical or population centers. On these bases, it is easy to understand why therapy for acquired adult articulation disorders is in its infancy. Without a clear understanding of the nature and natural course of these disorders, systematic design and evaluation of therapy interventions, including the optimal time to introduce them in the process of recovery or deterioration, is impossible. With the latest breakthroughs in instrumentation, and greater attention given to these disorders, the optimal data base defined in Figure 1-1 should be rapidly achieved, with a resultant improvement in accurate and early diagnosis and in the ultimate effectiveness of speech management.

REFERENCES

Barlow, S., and Abbs, J. (1983). Force transducers for the evaluation of labial, lingual, and mandibular motor impairments. *Journal of Speech and Hearing Research, 26,* 616–621.

Berry, W., Darley, F., Aronson, A., and Goldstein, N. (1973). Dysarthria in Wilson's disease. *Journal of Speech and Hearing Research, 17,* 169–183.

Beukelman, D., and Yorkston, K. (1977). A communication system for the severely dysarthric speaker with an intact language system. *Journal of Speech and Hearing Disorders, 42,* 265–270.

Birkmayer, W., and Hornykiewicz, O. (1961). Der L-3, 4-Dioxyohenylalanin (Dopa) effect bei der Parkinson akinese. *Wiener Klinische Wochenschrift, 73,* 787–799.

Blonsky, E., Logemann, J., Boshes, B., and Fisher, H. (1975). Comparison of speech and swallowing function in patients with tremor disorders and in normal geriatric patients: A cineradiographic study. *Journal of Gerontology, 30,* 299–303.

Blumstein, S., Cooper, W., Goodglass, H., Statlender, S., and Gottlieb, J. (1980). Production deficits in aphasia: A voice onset time analysis. *Brain and Language, 9,* 153–170.

Brodnitz, F. S. (1960). Speech after glossectomy. *Current Problems in Phoniatry and Logopedics, 1,* 68–72.

Brown, J., Darley, F., and Aronson, E. (1970). Ataxic dysarthria. *International Journal of Neurology, 7,* 302–318.

Burns, M., and Canter, G. (1977). Phonemic behavior of aphasic patients with posterior cerebral lesions. *Brain and Language, 4,* 492–507.

Calculator, S., and Dollaghan, C. (1982). The use of communication boards in residential setting: An evaluation. *Journal of Speech and Hearing Disorders, 47,* 281–287.

Canter, G. (1963). Speech characteristics of patients with Parkinson's disease: I. Intensity, pitch and duration. *Journal of Speech and Hearing Disorders, 28,* 221–229.

Canter, G. (1965a). Speech characteristics of patients with Parkinson's disease: II. Physiological support for speech. *Journal of Speech and Hearing Disorders, 30,* 44–49. (a)

Canter, G. (1965b). Speech characteristics of patients with Parkinson's disease: III. Articulation, diadochokinesis and overall speech adequacy. *Journal of Speech and Hearing Disorders, 30,* 217–224. (b)

Canter, G. (1964). Neuromotor pathologies of speech. *American Journal of Physical Medicine, 46,* 659–666.

Cantor, R., Curtis, T., Shipp, T., Beumer, J., and Vogel, B. (1969). Maxillary speech prostheses for mandibular surgical defects. *Journal of Prosthetic Dentistry, 22,* 253-257.

Coleman, C., Cook, A., and Meyers, L. (1980). Assessing nonoral clients for assistive communication devices. *Journal of Speech and Hearing Disorders, 45,* 515-526.

Copeland, K. (1974). *Aids for the severely handicapped.* New York: Grune & Stratton.

Critchley, E. (1981). Speech disorders of parkinsonism: A review. *Journal of Neurology, Neurosurgery, and Psychiatry, 44,* 751-758.

Daniel, B., and Guitar, B. (1978). EMG feedback and recovery of facial and speech gestures following neural anastomosis. *Journal of Speech and Hearing Disorders, 43,* 9-20.

Darley, F., Aronson, A., and Brown, J. (1968). Motor speech signs in neurologic disease. *Medical Clinics of North America, 52,* 840-844.

Darley, F., Aronson, A., and Brown, J. (1969). Differential diagnostic patterns of dysarthria. *Journal of Speech and Hearing Research, 12,* 462-496.

Darley, F., Aronson, A., and Brown, J. (1975). *Motor speech disorders.* Philadelphia: W. B. Saunders.

Donaldson, R. C., Skelly, M., and Paletta, F. X. (1968). Total glossectomy for cancer. *American Journal of Surgery, 116,* 585-590.

Drane, J. B. (1973). Prosthetic considerations in oral ablative surgery. *ASHA Reports, 8,* 39-41.

Duguay, M. J. (1964). Speech after glossectomy. *New York Journal of Medicine, 64,* 1836-1838.

Dworkin, J., and Hartman, D. (1979). Progressive speech deterioration and dysphagia in amyotrophic lateral sclerosis: Case report. *Archives of Physical Medicine and Rehabilitation, 60,* 423-425.

Fairbanks, G. (1958). *Voice and articulation drillbook.* New York: Harper.

Farmakides, M., and Boone, D. (1970). Speech problems of patients with multiple sclerosis. *Journal of Speech and Hearing Disorders, 25,* 385-390.

Georgian, D., Logemann, J., and Fisher, H. (1982). Compensatory articulation patterns of a patient after 20% glossectomy. *Journal of Speech and Hearing Disorders, 47,* 77-82.

Hand, C., Burns, M., and Ireland, E. (1979). Treatment of hypertonicity in muscles of lip retraction. *Biofeedback and Self Regulation, 4,* 171-181.

Hanson, W., and Metter, E. (1980). DAF as instrumental treatment for dysarthria in progressive supranuclear palsy: A case report. *Journal of Speech and Hearing Disorders, 45,* 268-276.

Hardy, J. (1965). Air flow and air pressure studies. *ASHA Reports, No. 1,* 141-152.

Herberman, M. A. (1958). Rehabilitation of patients following glossectomy. *Archives of Otolaryngology, 67,* 182-183.

Hirose, H. (1978). Electromyography of the articulatory muscles: Current instrumentation and technique. *Haskins Laboratory Status Reports on Speech Research, SR 25/26,* 73-85.

Hirose, H., Kiritani, S., Ushijima, T., and Sawashima, M. (1978). Analysis of abnormal articulatory dynamics in two dysarthric patients. *Journal of Speech and Hearing Disorders, 43,* 96-105.

Itoh, M., Sasanuma, S., Hirose, H., Yoshioka, H., and Ushijima, T. (1980). Abnormal articulatory dynamics in a patient with apraxia of speech: X-ray microbeam observation. *Brain and Language, 11,* 66-75.

Iwata, S., von Leden, H., and Williams, D. (1972). Air flow measurement during phonation. *Journal of Communication Disorders, 5,* 67-69.

Joanette, Y., and Dudley, J. (1980). Dysarthric symptomatology of Friedreich's ataxia. *Brain and Language, 10,* 39-50.

Johns, D., and Darley, F. (1970). Phonemic variability in apraxia of speech. *Journal of Speech and Hearing Research, 14,* 131-143.

Kent, R., and Netsell, R. (1975). A case study of an ataxic dysarthric: Cineradiographic and spectrographic observation. *Journal of Speech and Hearing Disorders, 40,* 115–134.

Kent, R., Netsell, R., and Abbs, J. (1979). Acoustic characteristics of dysarthria associated with cerebellar disease. *Journal of Speech and Hearing Research, 22,* 627–648.

Kiritani, S., Ito, K., and Fujimura, O. (1975). Tongue-pellet tracking by a computer controlled x-ray microbeam system. *Journal of the Acoustic Society of America, 57,* 1516–1520.

La Pointe, L., and Johns, D. (1975). Some phonemic characteristics in apraxia of speech. *Journal of Communication Disorders, 8,* 259–269.

Lazarus, C., and Logemann, J. (1982, November). *Compensatory articulation patterns in a 70% glossectomee.* Paper presented at the Annual Convention of the American Speech-Language-Hearing Association, Toronto.

Leanderson, R., Meyerson, B., and Persson, A. (1972). Lip muscle function in parkinsonian dysarthria. *Acta Otolaryngologica, 74,* 271–278.

Lehiste, I. (1968). *Some acoustic characteristics of dysarthria.* Basel: S. Karger.

Lehman, W., Hulicka, I., and Mehringer, E. (1966). Prosthetic treatment following complete glossectomy. *Journal of Prosthetic Dentistry, 16,* 344–350.

Leonard, R., and Gillis, R. (1982). Effects of a prosthetic tongue on vowel intelligibility and food management in a patient with total glossectomy. *Journal of Speech and Hearing Disorders, 47,* 25–30.

Linebaugh, C. (1979). The dysarthrias of Shy-Drager syndrome. *Journal of Speech and Hearing Disorders, 44,* 55–60.

Linebaugh, C., Baird, J., Baird, C., and Armour, R. (1983). Special considerations for the development of microcomputer based augmentative communication systems. In W. Berry (Ed.), *Clinical dysarthria.* San Diego: College-Hill Press.

Logemann, J., Boshes, B., Blonsky, E., and Fisher, H. (1977). Speech and swallowing evaluation in the differential diagnosis of neurologic disease. *Neurologia, Neurochirigia, Psychiatria, 18,* 71–78.

Logemann, J., Boshes, B., and Fisher, H. (1973). The steps in the degeneration of speech and voice control in Parkinson's disease. In J. Siegried (Ed.), *Parkinson's disease.* Vienna: Hans Huber.

Logemann, J., and Bytell, D. (1978, November). *Articulation patterns of five groups of head and neck surgical patients.* Paper presented at the Annual Convention of the American Speech and Hearing Association, San Francisco.

Logemann, J., and Bytell, D. (1979). Swallowing disorders in three types of head and neck surgical patients. *Cancer, 44,* 1095–1105.

Logemann, J., and Fisher, H. (1981). Vocal tract control in Parkinson's disease: Phonetic feature analysis of misarticulations. *Journal of Speech and Hearing Disorders, 46,* 348–352.

Logemann, J. A., Fisher, H., Boshes, B., and Blonsky, E. (1978). Frequency and cooccurrence of vocal tract dysfunctions in the speech of a large sample of Parkinson patients. *Journal of Speech and Hearing Disorders, 43,* 47–57.

Logemann, J., Fisher, H., and Bytell, D. (1977, November). *Functional effects of reconstruction in partially glossectomized patients.* Paper presented at the Annual Convention of the American Speech and Hearing Association, Chicago.

Logemann, J., Sisson, G., and Wheeler, R. (1980). The team approach to rehabilitation of surgically treated oral cancer patients. *Proceedings of the National Forum on Cancer Rehabilitation,* 222–227, Williamsburg, VA, November 13–15.

Ludlow, C., and Bassich, C. (1982). The results of acoustic and perceptual assessment of two types of dysarthria. In W. Berry (Ed.), *Clinical dysarthria.* San Diego: College-Hill Press.

Lybolt, J., Netsell, R., and Farrage, J. (1982, November). *A bite-block prosthesis in the treatment of dysarthria*. Paper presented at the Annual Convention of the American Speech-Language-Hearing Association, Toronto.

Mackay, R. (1963). Course and prognosis in amyotrophic lateral sclerosis. *Archives of Neurology, 8*, 117-127.

Mawdesley, C. (1973). Speech in parkinsonism. In D. Calne (Ed.), *Advances in neurology 3: Progress in the treatment of parkinsonism*. London: Raven.

McConnell, F. (1982, April). *Effects of surgical reconstruction on speech after oral ablative surgery*. Paper presented at the American Academy of Head and Neck Surgery, New Orleans.

McDonald, E., and Schultz, A. (1973). Communication boards for cerebral palsied children. *Journal of Speech and Hearing Disorders, 38*, 73-88.

Meyerson, B. (1973). EMG characteristics of labial articulatory muscles in parkinsonism. In J. Siegfried (Ed.), *Parkinson's disease*. Vienna: Hans Huber.

Montgomery, J. (1983). Communication systems for the child without speech. In W. Perkins (Ed.), *Dysarthria and apraxia*. New York: Thieme Stratton.

Moore, D. (1972). Glossectomy rehabilitation by mandibular tongue prosthesis. *Journal of Prosthetic Dentistry, 28*, 429-434.

Nakano, K., Zubick, H., and Tyler, H. (1973). Speech defects in parkinsonian patients. *Neurology, 23*, 865-870.

Netsell, R., and Cleeland, C. (1973). Modification of lip hypertonia in dysarthria using EMG feedback. *Journal of Speech and Hearing Disorders, 38*, 131-140.

Netsell, R., and Daniel, B. (1979). Dysarthria in adults: Physiologic approach to rehabilitation. *Archives of Physical Medicine and Rehabilitation, 60*, 502-508.

Netsell, R., Daniel, B., and Celesia, C. (1975). Acceleration and weakness in parkinsonian dysarthrias. *Journal of Speech and Hearing Disorders, 40*, 467-480.

Netsell, R., and Hixon, T. (1978). Noninvasive method for clinically estimating subglottal air pressure. *Journal of Speech and Hearing Disorders, 43*, 326-330.

Owens, R., and House, L. (1984). Decision-making processes in augmentative communication. *Journal of Speech and Hearing Disorders, 49*, 18-45.

Peacher, W. (1947). Speech disorders in World War II: VII. Treatment of dysarthrias. *Journal of Nervous and Mental Diseases, 106*, 66-76.

Peacher, W. (1950). The etiology and differential diagnosis of dysarthria. *Journal of Speech and Hearing Disorders, 15*, 252-265.

Rigrodsky, S., and Morrison, E. (1970). Speech changes in parkinsonism during L-Dopa therapy: Preliminary findings. *Journal of the American Geriatric Society, 18*, 142-151.

Rubow, R., Rosenbek, J., Collins, M., and Celesia, G. (1984). Reduction of hemifacial spasm and dysarthria following EMG biofeedback. *Journal of Speech and Hearing Disorders, 49*, 26-33.

Schweiger, J., Netsell, R., and Sommerfield, R. (1970). Prosthetic management and speech improvement in individuals with dysarthria of the palate. *Journal of the American Dental Association, 80*, 1348-1353.

Seilo, M. T., LaRiviere, C., and Dommick, K. C. (1972). *Report on the speech intelligibility of a glossectomee: Perceptual and acoustic observations*. Paper presented at the Annual Convention of the American Speech and Hearing Association, San Francisco.

Shane, H., and Bashir, A. (1980). Election criteria for the adoption of an augmentative communication system: Preliminary considerations. *Journal of Speech and Hearing Disorders, 45*, 408-414.

Silverman, F. (1983). Dysarthria: Communication-augmentation systems for adults without speech. In W. Perkins (Ed.), *Dysarthria and apraxia*. New York: Thieme-Stratton.

Skelly, M., Donaldson, R., and Fust, R. (1973). Glossectomee speech rehabilitation, Springfield, IL: Charles C Thomas.

Skelly, M., Donaldson, R., Fust, R., and Townsend, D. (1972). Changes in phonatory aspects of glossectomee intelligibility through vocal parameter manipulation. *Journal of Speech and Hearing Disorders, 37,* 379-389.

Skelly, M., Schinsky, L., Smith, R., and Fust, R. (1974). American Indian sign (Amerind) as a facilitator of verbalization for the oral verbal apraxic. *Journal of Speech and Hearing Disorders, 39,* 445-456.

Skelly, M., Spector, D., Donaldson, R., Brodeur, and Paletta, F. (1971). Compensatory physiologic phonetics for the glossectomee. *Journal of Speech and Hearing Disorders, 35,* 101-114.

Sonies, B. (1982). Oral imaging systems: A review and clinical applications. The *Journal of the National Student Speech Language Hearing Association, 10,* 30-43.

Sonies, B., Shauker, T., and Stowe, M. (1982, November). *Frontiers in oral imaging: Instrumentation and clinical application.* Paper presented at the Annual Convention of the American Speech-Language-Hearing Association, Toronto.

Summers, G. W. (1974). Physiologic problems following ablative surgery of the head and neck. *Otolaryngologic Clinics of North America, 7,* 217-250.

Trost, J., and Canter, G. (1974). Apraxia of speech in patients with Broca's aphasia: A study of phoneme production accuracy and error patterns. *Brain and Language, 1,* 63-80.

Vanderheiden, G., and Grilley, K. (Eds.) (1976). *Nonvocal communication techniques and aids for the severely physically handicapped.* Baltimore: University Park Press.

Vanderheiden, G., Kelso, D., Holt, C., and Raitzer, G. (1977). Development of flexible teacher-modifiable communication aids for the severely and extremely motor impaired. *Proceedings of the 4th Annual Conference on Systems and Devices for the Disabled* (pp. 86-91). Seattle: University of Washington.

Wertz, R., LaPointe, L., and Rosenbek, J. (1984). *Apraxia of speech in adults.* Orlando, FL: Grune & Stratton.

Wheeler, R., Logemann, J., and Rosen, M. (1980). Maxillary reshaping prostheses: Effectiveness in improving speech and swallowing of post-surgical oral cancer patients. *Journal of Prosthetic Dentistry, 43,* 313-319.

Chapter 2

Some Motor Control Perspectives on Apraxia of Speech and Dysarthria

James H. Abbs and
John C. Rosenbek

In our approaches to speech neuropathologies over the last 30 years, we have acquired certain methods, concepts, and definitions. For example, speech errors in dysarthria and apraxia of speech populations have been classified with the same schemes used for distinguishing the languages of the world. Likewise, descriptive techniques from experimental phonetics (e.g., perceptual, acoustic, and aerodynamic analyses) have been applied. Speech pathologists have also become involved in a number of theoretic issues, such as the "level" of these neural dysfunctions in relation to the phonetician's classic, multilayer analogy of the the speech production process. One example of such an issue is whether apraxia of speech is a disorder at the linguistic or the motor level. Many of these particular lines of description and theory appear, in part, to be historical accidents; current approaches to speech neuropathologies emerged from linguistics, experimental phonetics, and the educational and behavioral sciences. Accident or not, they have influenced the profession's perspective on theoretic and practical issues.

While some of the inheritance from these traditional antecedents has been useful, there is a danger of being misguided like the proverbial blind men in their exploration of the elephant. That is, if the attempt is to understand and treat human speech problems as breakdowns in social interaction or as loss of abstract symbol systems used for communication, such behavioral and linguistic approaches may, by themselves, be adequate. However, if by contrast the attempt is to understand the causal relations between certain brain dysfunctions and the programming, execution, and control of speech movements, equal emphasis must be placed upon the neurophysiology of motor control. The inclusion of current knowledge from motor control (as this area currently is defined [cf. Brooks, 1981]) requires careful consideration of the complex and flexible nature of motorsensory processes. As a bonus, the investigator becomes sensitive to the limitations of traditional concepts and analyses developed originally in experimental phonetics for other purposes.

The degree of imbalance in current approaches to speech neuropathologies is reflected in the nearly exclusive use of acoustic, aerodynamic, or perceptual analyses to discern the movement patterns of the vocal organs, seemingly as a basis upon which to make subsequent inferences regarding function and dysfunction of the nervous system. For example, acoustic signals are interpreted via models of vocal tract resonance that assume a general linear relation between vocal behavior and certain signal parameters. Paradoxically, little or no parallel consideration is given to the even more complex and nonlinear properties of muscle contraction, biomechanics, motor unit recruitment, and so on. This omission is particularly striking because neurophysiologic data indicate that determining moment-to-moment nervous system actions is exceedingly difficult even when the motor behaviors (movement and muscle activity) are observed directly (cf. Alexander, 1981; Partridge and Benton, 1981). Hence, as noted, these neurophysiologic considerations bring into sharp focus the parallel ambiguity in discerning motor-sensory operation from the far less direct acoustic, aerodynamic, or auditory-perceptual analyses. For these and other reasons to be discussed, a neuromotor control approach is needed to augment and verify traditional analyses and to provide a more rational perspective for considering these disorders in both the laboratory and the clinic. That is, while traditional methods from experimental phonetics are accepted within speech pathology, and many practitioners are "comfortable" with their use, a broader approach to dysarthria and apraxia is likely, in the long run, to provide a fundamental basis for sustaining future progress.

In this context, the purpose of this chapter is to offer some alternative interpretations on the nature, evaluation, and management of dysarthria and apraxia of speech from a state-of-the-art neuroscience perspective. Throughout this presentation, it is our hope to raise questions and offer information that will stimulate future research and new ideas on these particular disorders. Some of our notions are speculative, but they are included to provoke debate and to illustrate the equally speculative nature of some of the current "plausible" hypotheses. It should be noted that this chapter is not intended to be a review of all recent research on dysarthria and apraxia of speech. Nor is our goal to provide specific information that can be translated immediately into clinical activities; we will be encouraged if that happens. Rather, the primary objective is to provide a catalyst for a more direct focus upon the actual functions and dysfunctions of the nervous system. In parallel, we hope to retain those aspects of our earlier knowledge that remain useful, while discarding baggage we have acquired in traveling on some dead end roads.

RATIONALE FOR A MOTOR CONTROL APPROACH

In attempting to study, diagnose, or treat dysarthria and apraxia of speech, our fundamental objective is to address problems in the nervous system programming and execution of speech movements. While we admit to the general accuracy of the platitudes suggesting that speech is one of the human's most "complex" motor behaviors, it is undeniable that speech production is nevertheless a *motor act* with commonalities to other voluntary motor behavior in terms of muscle contractions, movements, biomechanics, motoneuron recruitment, and so on. As such, in the attempt to decipher nervous system function for speech production, it is useful to acknowledge and understand these common elements, thereby giving us at least an initial perspective on the complexities involved.

Table 2–1 is a list of the probable components of speech neuromotor programming and control, drawn from both contemporary neurophysiology and parallel knowledge of speech production processes. In the sequence from the acoustic signal output of the speech production system (level 1) to successively "deeper" levels of motor-sensory function (levels 3, 4, 5, etc.), it is apparent that several critical processes have not been considered carefully in analyses of speech motor control. For example, the way that motoneuron signals activate muscle actions (level 2) has alone been the subject of an estimated 100,000 reported investigations. Without knowledge of this critical link, inferences from peripheral to higher levels is fraught with potential error. Seldom, however, are any of the potential influences of muscle, the neuromotor end organ of the speech production system, considered even implicitly in interpretations of speech neuropathologies. It might be argued that the process of translating motoneuron signals to muscle contraction is a simple one, and hence a linear relation can be assumed. However, as noted recently by Partridge and Benton (1981) in their extensive review of muscle biomechanics research, "a number of

Table 2-1. Probable Biologic Processes Underlying "Significant" Speech Production Features

1. *Acoustic and aerodynamic properties of the vocal conduit,* including physical discontinuities or nonlinearities

2. *Biomechanical properties,* e.g., muscle mechanics, load dynamics, geometric nonlinearities, boundary conditions

3. *Lower level reflexive actions,* via lower brainstem or spinal cord pathways

4. *Modifiable, long-loop reactions* (transcortical cerebellar-cerebral, etc.), possibly developed or refined with experience

5. *Internal CNS refinement and predictive correction processes,* variably dependent on moment-to-moment ascending afferents

6. *Sets of general, prelearned motor goals,* as a basis for overall guidance of CNS execution and programming

7. *Linguistic specification of "segmental" or suprasegmental goals,* as currently hypothesized or as yet undefined

or, most likely,

8. *Variable and awesomely complex interactions among all levels of this biolinguistic process*

models exist that approximate parts of muscle function, but all of the models inescapably have appreciable defects. Deficiencies lie in both the formal models available and in defects in our understanding of the rules of the biological muscle as it responds to mechanical and neural actions" (p. 47). In short, Partridge and Benton indicate that our current knowledge does not, except under restricted circumstances, allow us to understand the seemingly simple relation between motoneuron firing patterns and movement, to say nothing of inferring in the opposite direction (i.e., from movement to nervous system actions).

Similarly, in noting the potential role of the primary sensory and motor cortices to the control of movement, Evarts (1981), while documenting the involvement of a transcortical feedback pathway, offers a number of plausible, yet tentative, hypotheses concerning the actual function of that pathway and its peripheral sensory motor correlates. Given the complex, multiple levels of motor programming and control (see Table 2-1), it is critical to consider the undeniable contributions of these various processes to the relatively superficial events we are able to observe at the speech production periphery. In other words, for any apparently significant normal or abnormal feature of the speech production output, be it perceptually, acoustically, aerodynamically, or electromyographically detected, we cannot, without being extremely careful, talk about the nervous system origins of that feature. What should be apparent from these comments is that the surface analysis procedures we are able to apply to neurologically impaired speech production systems are likely to yield indices of dysfunction that are "an awesomely complex and variable combination of all levels of this biolinguistic process" (see Table 2-1). However, despite this caution, it is possible, based upon the substantial and largely ignored literature on motor neurophysiology, to extend and critically examine our current notions concerning the nature, assessment, and treatment of speech neuropathologies.

Also of particular value in this effort is the emergence in the last ten years of clinical neurophysiology. Clinical neurophysiology (as a subspecialty of neurology) has the following goals: (1) to provide a quantitative profile of the neurologic signs and performance deficits with which to diagnose, prescribe, and evaluate treatment; (2) to relate these disease-associated indices to working models of the normal and neurologically impaired nervous system; and (3) to examine these profiles of the nervous system to identify and test hypotheses that might point to improved programs of assessment and treatment (cf. Stalberg and Young, 1981). From this effort, the size of which is illustrated by several volumes of clinical neurophysiology research edited by one scholar (Desmedt, 1973-1982), has come a data base upon which to consider current approaches to the nervous system dysfunctions underlying apraxia of speech and dysarthria. While consideration of all the potential implications of clinical neurophysiology and motor control for speech neuropathologies is outside the scope of this chapter, the data and sources cited should provided a basis for parallel review and synthesis efforts by most readers.

From the standpoint of what might be gained from acknowledging the limitations of certain current perspectives on speech neuropathologies, we should like to borrow a quote from motor neurophysiologist and Nobel Laureate Ragnar Granit (1977): "In dealing with objects of our research whose explanation from the standpoint of present-day science is insufficient, greater scientific clarity is achieved by fully realizing what cannot be explained than by stealing a march on science with suppositions. We cannot reach further than to understand what can be understood and realize what we cannot understand" (p. 1). To paraphrase, if we don't know where we really are now, how can we make intelligent decisions on how to get where we want to go?

THE DISTINCTION BETWEEN DIAGNOSIS AND ASSESSMENT: THE CRITICAL USE OF DESCRIPTIVE TERMS

In the discussions that follow, at least an implicit emphasis will be placed upon examining the current semantics of dysarthria and apraxia of speech, and the degree to which these terms, in and of themselves, become issues, often without a substantive foundation. In this vein, it appears important to consider the categorizing processes involved in accomplishing our clinical objectives and ask what the conventional labels and terms do and do not provide.

It has been common to distinguish the different neuropathologies of speech via contrastive profiles of descriptive behaviors. One common difficulty, in neurology as well as speech pathology, has been the assumption that these diagnostic indicators of a particular neuropathologic syndrome are coincident with or underlie the debilitating performance deficits associated with the disease. For example, in the person with spastic dysarthria, it has been assumed that some of the diagnostically distinct speech signs can be ascribed to hypertonicity in the form of muscle spasms. The so-called "strained-strangled voice" observed in these dysarthric persons is thought to be due to antagonistic or spastic co-contraction of the intrinsic laryngeal muscles. In this example, the term spasticity has been borrowed from neurology, and further assumptions have been made that this manifestation of the motor disorder in the limbs is present also in the laryngeal muscles, and that "spasticity," per se, is a causal factor in the speech disorder. To the knowledge of the present authors, muscle activity in the intrinsic laryngeal muscles has not been observed in a classic case of spastic dysarthria; that is, the suggestion of spastic hypertonicity is conjecture. Additionally, it is not clear, even to the clinical neurophysiologists who have spent their careers attempting to quantify and treat spasticity, how best to define it (cf. Lance, 1980; Landau, 1980). For example, is spasticity exclusively a velocity-dependent increase in stretch reflexes, causing a pathophysiologic increase in resistance to a neurologic examiner's externally imposed movement? Or, as suggested by some, is it synonymous with the so-called upper motoneuron syndrome involving decreased dexterity, loss of strength, increased tendon jerks, increased resistance to passive stretch, and hyperactive flexion reflexes? It is apparent that spasticity is not a unidimensional phenomenon. Perhaps most critical to this example is the current consensus among experimental and clinical neurologists that while spasticity, per se, is an excellent diagnostic sign, the increased hypertonus-hyperactive stretch reflex-flexor spasms seen in these patients are largely independent from the actual motor performance deficits present in parallel. Landau (1980) was particularly candid and clear in reviewing several lines of evidence (Denny-Brown, 1980; Duncan, Shahani, and Young, 1976; Landau, 1974, 1980; Sahrman and Norton, 1977) concerning the relation between hypertonic signs and motor performance impairments in spastic patients. He noted, "However useful to clinical diagnosis may be the increase of excitability at anterior horn cells and to some extent muscle spindles, these phenomena have little more relation to the patient's disability than does the insertion of the rectal thermometer in pneumonia" (p. 20). In this context, one must seriously question the assertion that so-called strained-strangled voice is the result of antagonistic muscle "spastic" hypertonus in the larynx.

There is obviously a very important message in this example for the distinction between diagnosis and assessment. That is, while it is logical and intuitively appealing to make the inference that hypertonus and spasms are the *major underlying cause* of motor disabilities in persons with spasticity or upper motoneuron syndrome, this inference does not stand up to empirical scrutiny. Indeed, this unfounded assumption was made by both clinical and research neurophysiologists over the years, and millions of dollars were spent on attempts to eliminate hypertonus with the expectation that the motor deficit associated with this disorder would be improved in parallel. As noted by Landau (1980), these results have been disappointing.

It is also likely that some of the most salient distinguishing indicators for differential diagnosis of these speech neuropathologies may not be related causally to the speech performance deficits that are present in parallel. That is, in the use of traditional techniques from experimental phonetics, or even so-called physiologic measures, examination must be made of the extent to which certain acoustic, aerodynamic, auditory-perceptual, or electromyographic features of speech "abnormality" are related *causally* to deficits in functional communication or speech movement coordination and control. Certainly, it would seem a minimal scientific requirement that such descriptive analyses focus upon measures that are correlated to the degree of functional speech disturbance. Correlational analyses, without analytic models or explicit hypotheses for verifying causality, are highly subject to misinterpretation. However, these data, at the least, would assist us in determining what aspects of performance aberration are epiphenomena, and hence of minor significance, and at the same time identify those aberrant features that might reflect overall performance deficits. If we adhere to these requirements in our research and treatment, we might avoid repeating the errors made in the attempted treatment of spasticity and also enhance the rational basis for focusing our programs of rehabilitation. To return to the example of limb spasticity discussed earlier, it is apparent that reducing or eliminating flexor spasms or hyperactive stretch reflexes through various treatments was not of particular benefit in improving motor function. Treating certain superficial aberrations (e.g., acoustic segment durations) may be similarly futile unless such aberrations have been demonstrated as negative neurologic manifestations and not simply epiphenomena. The message is clear. The seemingly compelling causal relations that might be observed in clinical populations may not be valid; the nervous system often does not function in intuitively obvious ways, and the requirement for formal testing of unquantified assertions, no matter how appealing they may be, cannot be relaxed. The penalty for an absence of seemingly harsh empiricism in clinical endeavors is ineffective treatment.

CONCEPTUALIZATION OF THE SPEECH MOTOR CONTROL PROCESS

As noted at the outset of this chapter, certain extant models of the speech production process appear to have had considerable impact upon our conceptualization of speech neuropathologies, and thus upon the way in which these disorders are assessed, treated, and studied. One such "model," either implicitly or explicitly incorporated in most thinking about normal and disordered speech production systems, portrays the speech production process as a succession of independent levels proceeding from semantic, to syntactic, to phonologic formulations. Phonetic goals are achieved via the seemingly mechanical operation of motor programming and execution. Such representations may be quite functional if the issues addressed are in the domain of psycholinguistics. However, this representation carries with it certain simplifying assumptions, which may be counterproductive in our approaches to dysarthria and apraxia of speech. One of these assumptions is that intended phonologic-phonetic goals yield stereotyped and consistent muscle activities, movements, and vocal tract shapes at the periphery. More specifically, this model implies that once a string of phonetic goals is specified, the "lower levels" of this process involve the more or less direct activation of a set of muscle actions. Further, it is implied that the set of muscle actions is essentially the same every time a particular phonetic string is produced. This conceptualization implies a single, isolated level of motor programming, and hence the execution process is conceived primarily as the transmission of temporally-spatially correct signals to the periphery.

In the context of numerous recent experiments on these motor programming, coordination, and execution processes, this view (or the subtle variations on it presented in many accounts of speech production) is simply not tenable. That is, in the last decade we have seen an exponential increase in the research efforts on voluntary motor control; it has been estimated that 500 papers per month are published in this area (Partridge, 1976). Hence, on the basis of this intensive application of new techniques to discern the character of nervous system function in movement control (cf. Desmedt, 1978 [1973–1982]; Houk and Rymer, 1981; Rack, 1981, for reviews), extensive evidence indicates that speech motor programming and execution cannot be characterized in this traditional manner. As Marsden (1982) noted recently in regard to motor execution:

> in the real world, such admittedly central motor programs are never isolated from peripheral feedback which must operate at all stages in the sequence of a motor act. Computing technology has introduced the concept of hierarchic schemes that greatly simplify and shorten the programming of robot manipulations. Such systems, remarkably reminiscent of the various levels of Hughlings Jackson, utilize different levels of control, each one of which regulates its own particular function or parameter. The levels of control are arranged in hierarchic order, the more general subordinating and modulating the more specific. Each level receives information about the state of the other levels. In practice, the entire hierarchical system operates as a whole to produce an integrated, smooth performance. (p. 523)

While this observation is based upon experiments conducted on limb motor behavior in man and waking animals, parallel observations in the speech production system suggest qualitatively similar principles of motor programming and execution. For example, inasmuch as programming and associated descending signals appear to be under continual modulation and updating via ascending afferent information, it is apparent that the generation of a given articulatory movement or vocal tract shape is not prespecified stereotypically, but rather varies from one production of a given utterance to a repeated production of that same utterance. This is indeed what has been observed empirically. Hughes and Abbs (1976) transduced the movements of the upper lip, lower lip, and jaw during repeated productions of a particular utterance. The classic model discussed earlier would predict, within certain system noise limits, that these articulators would move essentially in the same way for these repeated productions. However, when the actual movements were observed for multiple repetitions of the same utterance, there was not a stereotypic pattern. For a given repetition, when the jaw moved a large distance in producing an oral opening for a vowel, the upper and lower lips moved a small distance; for another repetition, the relative magnitude of movement between these coordinated structures was reversed. More specifically, the normal motor control of the oral opening was not achieved in a stereotypic manner, but rather involved a considerable degree of repetition-to-repetition trade-off between movements of these three contributing articulators. Similar trade-offs have been reported between the tongue and the jaw (Fujimura, 1981) and the rib cage and abdomen (Hunker and Abbs, 1982). Further observations have been made indicating that two synergistic muscles that contribute to the movement of a given structure likewise trade off in their contributions from one generation of that movement to another, both in the limbs (Lacquaniti and Soechting, 1982) and in the speech production system (Abbs, 1979; Abbs and Gracco, 1984; Gentil, Gracco, and Abbs, 1983; Sussman, MacNeilage, and Hanson, 1973). Specifically, these latter observations indicate that two synergistic muscles that contribute to movement of a given structure (e.g., orbicularis oris inferior and mentalis in their conjoint contribution to lower lip elevation) are not activated stereotypically but trade off in the repetition-to-repetition generation of the same movement (Abbs, 1979; Abbs and Gracco, 1984).

Figure 2-1 provides a concrete, albeit simplified, example of these variations for three productions of the utterance /aba/ that were equivalent in terms of their phonologic, aerodynamic, acoustic, and auditory-perceptual characteristics. The upper and lower lip movements for these productions are shown, illustrating three different patterns of movement. Obviously, the muscle activity underlying these productions is different as well; essentially, this example illustrates complementary variation between upper and lower lip gestures to carry out an equivalent phonologic plan of action.

These observations on normal speech motor programming and execution are consistent with the comments made by Marsden and may require certain modifications in the traditional model presented earlier and in terms of the way speech pathologists have conceptualized the neuropathologies of speech. Initially, it is apparent that the motor execution and programming of speech is not a single operation, but a hierarchical process with considerable variation in the ways objectives and subobjectives are accomplished. That is, while the overall goals of the system output (e.g., oral opening, degree of oral constriction, subglottal pressure) might be considered part of the general phonologic plan of action, the temporal-spatial implementation of these goals via multiple movements is apparently programmed at another level of the system. Indeed, it is apparent that there

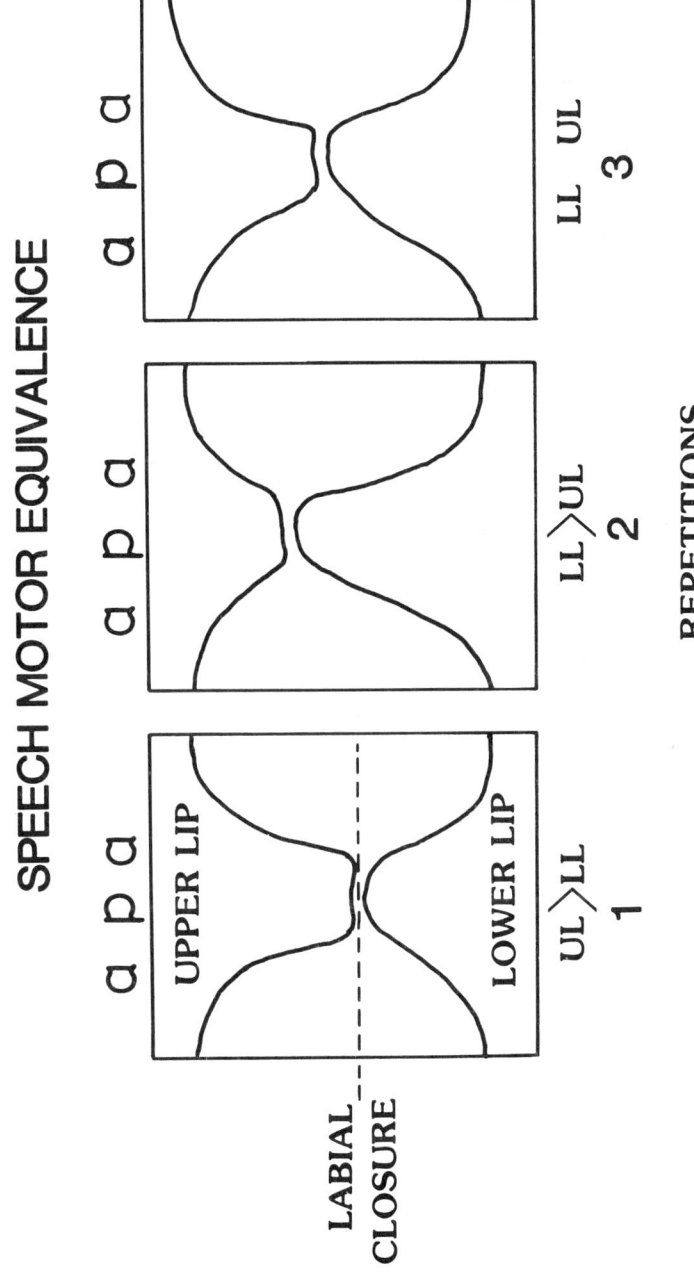

Figure 2-1. Upper and lower lip movements for a normal speaker for three repetitions of the utterance [apa]. In this example, the jaw was fixed with a bite-block.

is not a stereotypic or consistent relation between the movements of a given articulator and the hypothesized phonetic or phonologic goals. For example, production of a vowel with a narrow vocal tract opening does not require that the jaw be in a consistently high position, only that the combination of the jaw and the tongue together achieve this goal. Similar flexibility in the peripheral execution process apparently exists for relative contributions of the abdomen and rib cage to total lung volume or for contributions of the upper lip, lower lip, and jaw to oral opening and closing. Recent observations involving the introduction of small, unanticipated errors in lip movements suggest that this flexible, multimovement coordination process is accomplished via afferent ascending signals, possibly operating in a predictive manner (Abbs and Cole, 1982; Abbs and Gracco, 1982, 1984; Folkins and Abbs, 1975, 1976; Gracco and Abbs, 1982).

The observation of parallel trade-offs between synergistic muscles acting to achieve a particular movement further suggests that the neuromotor level where individual muscle actions are programmed is in turn separate from the level where individual movements are programmed. That is, the action of a particular muscle is not stereotyped for a given movement, but rather covaries, with other muscles also contributing to that movement from one repetition of the movement to another. Therefore, it is apparent that individual muscle contractions are at least two programming steps removed from the level of the nervous system where the so-called phonetic or overall goals are predetermined. Hence, the level of the nervous system where the so-called concept of action or the general motor plan is determined, perhaps involving phonologic goals, is different from the levels of motor programming where specific muscle contractions and movements are determined. In terms of our considerations of dysarthria and apraxia of speech, it is obvious that a useful approach involves questions concerning the possible neuromotor levels at which these problems are manifest. Because of the absence of a one-to-one correspondence between phonologic goals and motor outputs, it appears far less useful to attempt to separate motor dysfunctions from linguistic ones, especially with superficial peripheral measures. An intriguing issue regarding levels of programming concerns the distinction between oral, nonverbal apraxia, and apraxia of speech. Physiologic observations in these populations may reveal some additional distinctions concerning differences in the levels of motor programming for these behavioral deficits.

In addition to variations in individual movements and muscle contractions for repeated productions of the same utterance, there are parallel variations in overall vocal tract shapes for multiple productions of the same acoustic end product (Ladefoged, DeClark, Lindau, and Papcun, 1972; Lindau, Jacobson, and Ladefoged, 1972). All of these variations in movements, muscle contractions, and vocal tract shapes operate under the general principle of motor equivalence (cf. Bernstein, 1967; Hebb, 1949; Lacquaniti and Soechting, 1982; Lashley, 1930; Morasso, 1981). Motor equivalence is generally defined as a nervous system operation in which the same intended motor objective is accomplished with variation in the individual movements and muscle contractions that combine to produce that intended goal. This principle of motor control has particular implications for traditional experimental phonetic measures of speech neuropathologies. Initially, it is apparent that utterance productions judged equivalent by more global measures are likely to be very different in terms of underlying patterns of muscle activity, movement, or specific vocal tract configuration. The power of inferences made from these global measures to patterns of movement, muscle contraction, or nervous system activity in any but the most general terms is, therefore, very limited. For example, if the vocal tract acoustic transfer function underlying a particular vowel formant pattern requires certain vocal tract length characteristics or relative volumes of front and back cavities, these apparently are *not* produced in a stereotyped manner. Rather, they are produced through combinations of lip protrusion and laryngeal height for vocal tract length, and combinations of pharyngeal constriction–tongue body forwarding for front cavity–back cavity dimensions (Ladefoged et al., 1972; Lindau et al., 1972). Indeed, we have known for some time the substantial degrees of freedom available in the production of vowels (cf. Stevens and House, 1955, 1961, concerning covariable contributions of upper airway articulators). Similar variability is obviously available in the production of air pressures and air flow rates for speech, where manipulations in the upper airway size, shape, and cavity wall impedance, along with temporal-spatial variations in glottal abduction-adduction, allow for substantial degrees of freedom in the production of aerodynamically equivalent patterns (Muller and Brown, 1980).

In the same way, and perhaps to a greater extent, auditory-perceptual analyses, whether involving broad or narrow phonetic transcription, are subject to very serious limitations in the making of inferences to underlying movements and muscle contractions or specific moment-to-moment patterns of nervous system operation. We know from perceptual studies the degree to which speech acoustic signal cues can be varied and still remain acceptable in relation to phonetic categorization or from the standpoint of intelligibility. For example, the perceptual domain in /i/-ness is obviously not simply an absolute or relative formant frequency pattern; rather, it has perceptually significant acoustic features of duration, intensity, and fundamental frequency that have been shown to influence its identification. Inasmuch as these features apparently can be weighted relatively, especially in contextual speech, there appears to be a substantial possibility that perceptual equivalence is achieved, despite considerable idiosyncratic or compensatory acoustic variations (cf. Lindblom, 1982).

Given these potential sources of variation in the manner in which apparently equivalent productions (based upon acoustic, aerodynamic, or auditory-perceptual observations, or a combination thereof) are generated, it seems that in populations of disordered speakers known to invoke idiosyncratic compensatory adjustments, no single measure is adequate for inferences regarding underlying nervous system function or dysfunction. That is, these single measure analyses are, by definition, insensitive to the motor control equivalence variations. Moreover, that insensitivity is probably greatest where motor equivalence adjustments and maladjustments are employed with varying degrees of success in attempts to minimize the effects of nervous system abnormalities (Gracco and Muller, 1981; Nashner and Grimm, 1978).

This argument is supported, in part, by the general difficulty where global analyses have been employed in distinguishing among dysarthric subpopulations or between certain dysarthric and verbal apraxic groups. Practically every published analysis of the acoustic characteristics of dysarthric speech includes certain common features (e.g., increased vowel durations, inappropriate or lengthened pauses or both), despite known differences in the underlying neuropathophysiology. Similarly, when subjected to quantitative analyses, the numerous and long-standing attempts at auditory-perceptual distinctions between the speech of athetoid and spastic dysarthric persons reflect limited success, at best. The limited distinguishing capabilities of these global measures might be due to the fact that the nervous system has a finite set of compensation–motor equivalence adjustments. For example, some of these compensatory processes are likely to be invoked similarly by speakers with such conditions as cerebellar disease or apraxia of speech. Slowing of speech rate could be one such common strategy, despite rather substantial differences in the underlying neuropathophysiology. Further, when one is able, via global analyses, to distinguish the speech of two populations of patients with motor disorders, interpretations are further clouded. That is, the distinguishing features could reflect differences in compensatory capabilities and could be related only indirectly to primary motor performance deficits. In general, the implications of these considerations are that clinically we must attempt to observe the motor behavior of the speech production system under conditions where the complex and semiunpredictable normal and abnormal motor equivalence compensatory strategies are minimized. Given the limitations of observing the movements of all the speech structures during normal productions, this consideration, by necessity, translates to an argument for evaluations based upon simpler nonspeech gestures in parallel with our more traditional analyses. Most clinicians, of course, recognize this, at least implicitly, as is reflected in their use of the oral peripheral examination. Attempting to assess speech neuropathologies on the basis of speech behavior alone is comparable to asking our automobile mechanic to assess a malfunction in our automobile engine as we drive by on the interstate highway. Perhaps if we simplify our analyses, we can begin to focus rehabilitation on specific, less global motor malfunctions, and hence refine our approaches to these disorders. This argument, however, implies that nonspeech motor impairments are of value in assessing and managing motor speech disorders. This raises the classic issue of whether speech and nonspeech motor functions share a common underlying neural substrate.

HOW SPECIAL IS SPEECH?

A long-standing question in the assessment and treatment of motor speech disorders is related to two other questions. Do impairments in the motor control of nonspeech activities such as chewing and swallowing, or volitional nonspeech maneuvers (as observed in the oral peripheral examination), correlate with, or are they indicative of, parallel impairments in speech motor function? Further, does rehabilitation focused upon either feeding or nonspeech "voluntary" control of speech motor subsystems carry over, in its benefits, to improved speech control? Initially, it seems apparent that in lower motoneuron damage the carryover is likely to be high. That is, rehabilitation in the form of strengthening, if successful for nonspeech tasks, should yield improvements in speech as well. This issue, however, has been debated more intensely regarding speech motor problems resulting from supranuclear damage, either congenital or acquired.

Several lines of old and recent evidence are of particular relevance to this issue. Initially, it is important that speech and nonspeech motor tasks be defined from a current neurophysiologic perspective. Chewing, swallowing, and other orofacial vegetative functions are known to be neurophysiologically distinct from nonspeech tasks performed voluntarily. That is, it is documented that these vegetative functions are largely controlled via certain subcortical pattern generators, networks of brainstem reflexes, or both (cf. Dubner, Sessle, and Storey, 1978; Wyke, 1974). For example, Hoffman and Luschei (1980) demonstrated that while motor cortical activity was not involved in moment-to-moment control of chewing in rhesus monkeys, operantly conditioned biting (a "more voluntary" task using the same jaw muscles) was clearly under cortical influence. They noted, "a likely explanation for this observation is that the reciprocal action of the jaw closing and opening muscles during chewing is patterned elsewhere in the brain" (p. 342). Other recent work in the differential control of "automatic" and learned movements suggests a parallel dichotomy for the muscles of the respiratory system (Phillips and Porter, 1977) and the facial muscles (Denny-Brown, 1960). As noted recently by Evarts (1981):

> It might at first seem odd that corticospinal neurons controlling precise skilled movements terminate on motoneurons controlling intercostal muscles that participate in an act as automatic and primative as respiration, but Phillips and Porter point out that these terminations are probably related to the use of respiratory muscles in speech and song rather than in breathing. . . . Destroying the corticospinal projection to thoracic motoneurons does not impair the use of respiratory muscles for respiration, though these same muscles may be useless for speech. (p. 1113)

These considerations offer a new perspective on this long-standing controversy. That is, on the basis of current neurophysiologic observations, this issue does not appear to be one of speech versus nonspeech motor control. Rather, the critical distinction may be whether the nonspeech movements are controlled in a conscious, voluntary manner, as in speech, in contrast to vegetative movements that are more or less automatic. This interpretation appears to square with the data, both old and recent, that are available to address this issue. Perhaps the most concentrated effort in this area came in a series of master's theses conducted under the direction of James Hardy in the 1960s (Hixon, 1963; Murphy, 1966; Smit, 1969; Smith, 1964).

In these studies the relationship between several different orofacial speech tasks was examined in dysarthric subjects, and the results were interpreted with remarkable uniformity to indicate that speech "may well be dissimilar to other neuromuscular processes involving identical muscle groups" (Hardy, 1970, p. 60). In evaluation of these classic studies in light of the modified interpretation just offered, the motor task comparisons and correlations made must be examined carefully. The investigation reported by Hixon and Hardy (1964) is exemplary. Essentially, in this study independent indices were obtained for degree of speech severity, diadochokinetic rates for several different stop sounds, and rates of nonspeech voluntary movements such as lateral movements of the tongue. Degree of impairment in nonspeech vegetative movements such as chewing and swallowing was not reported. The results suggest fairly high correlations (0.70 to 0.75) between severity of speech and syllable diadochokinetic rates, and somewhat lower correlations between speech severity and rates of nonspeech movements (0.41 to 0.56).

The fundamental problem with Hixon and Hardy's study (1964) is that the comparison of these correlations does not support the interpretation of speech versus nonspeech control differences. The speech and the CV syllable diadochokinetic tasks obviously involved the respiratory system, larynx, and pharynx, as well as the tongue, lips, and jaw. By contrast, the tongue, lip, and jaw movements were sampled individually in the nonspeech movement tasks. Because the subject populations observed were probably variable in the degree of respiratory, laryngeal, and pharyngeal motor impairment, this would have the effect of reducing the correlations between severity of speech disorders and the rates of either lip, jaw, or tongue nonspeech movements. Recent data argue for ubiquitous differential speech subsystem impairment in patients with cerebral palsy and Parkinson's disease (cf. Abbs, Hunker, and Barlow, 1983; Barlow and Abbs, 1982; Hunker, Abbs, and Barlow, 1982). Indeed, given the near certainty of this contaminating factor, the correlations reported between individual articulator nonspeech movement rates and speech severity are relatively high; one of the present authors has actually cited these observations as support of an overlap between control processes for speech and nonspeech control (Abbs, Sutton, Larson, and Eilenberg, 1973). Another factor supporting an alternate interpretation for the Hixon and Hardy (1964) results was that the correlation between the degree of judged speech severity and the diadochokinetic rates for pVtVkV syllables (0.53) was in the same range as the correlations between judged speech severity and nonspeech movement rates. Additionally, the nonspeech movement that had the poorest correlation to speech severity (0.28) was raising the tongue to the aveolar ridge and lowering it, a maneuver that required a larger range of movement than for rapid production of diadochokinetic [da]s. By way of reinterpretation, the comparisons made in these often cited studies offer support, indirectly and directly, for a *common neuromuscular substrate* underlying control of speech and nonspeech *voluntary* tasks.

Direct evidence supporting a common neural substrate for the control of voluntary, nonspeech movements and speech are provided by instrumental observations of nonspeech control impairments of the tongue, lips, and jaw, and comparison of these measures with impairments in the movements of the same structures during speech (Barlow and Abbs, 1984; Hunker et al., 1982; Hunker and Abbs, 1984). Figure 2-2 shows a profile of nonspeech control impairment in a subject with congenital spasticity

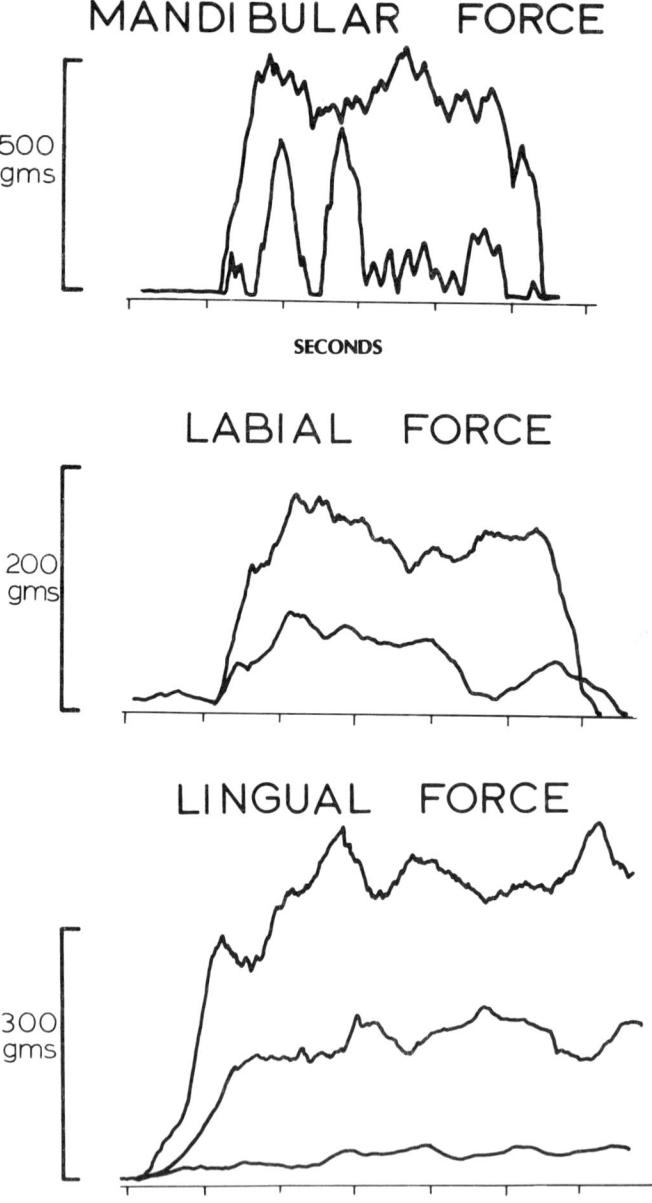

Figure 2-2. Comparison of fine force control of the lips, tongue, and jaw in a subject with congenital spasticity.

and dysarthria. As is apparent, the greatest degree of control impairment (with respect to normal performance) for this static force task was in the jaw; the lips and tongue were far less impaired. In this subject, a bite-block was placed between the teeth, effectively eliminating the need to control movement in the disproportionately impaired jaw. The result of the bite-block upon speech is shown in Figure 2–3, which contrasts the upper lip, lower lip, and jaw movements for conditions with the jaw free to vary and with the jaw fixed. Substantial improvements are apparent in the regularity of the upper and lower lip movements, intraoral air pressure (both magnitude and duration), and the durations and amplitudes of the vowels as reflected in the audio signal. These data are representative of those from a larger study, which demonstrated a high correlation (0.89) between degree of impairment in the voluntary, nonspeech control of the lips, jaw, and tongue, and measures of speech severity (Barlow and Abbs, 1984). Similarly, in a group of parkinsonian dysarthric subjects, Hunker and colleagues (1982) found a positive correlation between degree of labial rigidity, range of lip movement, and severity of dysarthria. In summary, these latter data and the previously considered neurophysiologic and neuroanatomic findings suggest that nonspeech control of precise, voluntary activities is likely to be impaired in the same manner as speech motor behavior.

The implications for assessment and rehabilitation from this working hypothesis are several. Initially, on the basis of the data shown in Figure 2–3, it is obvious that assessment of impairments solely on the basis of spontaneous speech behavior, whether movement observations, acoustic analyses, or simply a sage clinical ear is used, may not permit differentiation of a jaw control impairment from a lip or tongue impairment. These data from spastic and hypokinetic dysarthric subjects address an important point made previously regarding the relative insensitivity of more global indices provided by acoustic or aerodynamic analyses. Specifically, it is unlikely that without use of a bite-block the critical jaw control impairment in the spastic dysarthric subject would have been discernible from such measures as formant frequencies, vowel durations, and air pressure measures. Similarly, conventional global measures would not be sensitive to the differential degree of upper and lower lip rigidity in the parkinsonian dysarthric patients. Hence, observations of voluntary nonspeech control tasks obviously are useful to separate potential subsystem motor impairments. This logic carries over to rehabilitation as well. That is, if impairments of voluntary nonspeech control are parallel to those for speech, improvements on selected, voluntary nonspeech tasks could be expected to enhance speech control as well, depending of course on the site of the lesion and neural tissue remaining to support voluntary and learned behaviors. Thus, for the rehabilitation of the spastic dysarthric subject

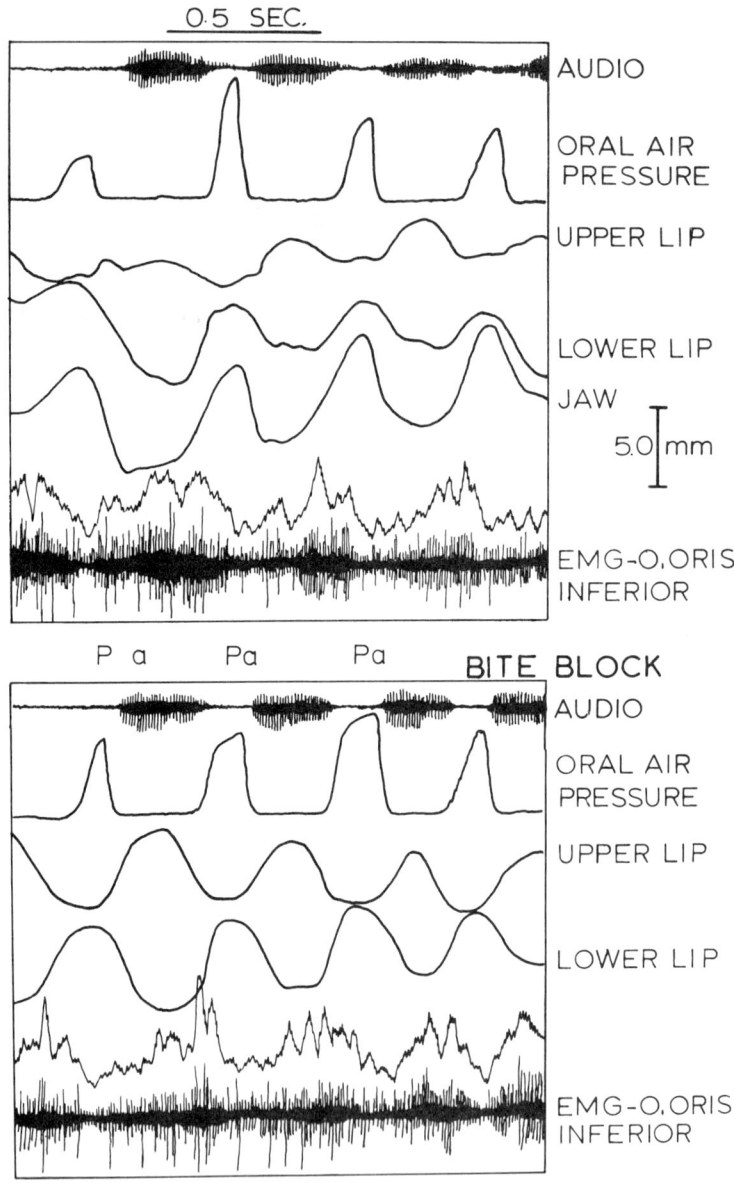

Figure 2-3. Comparison of labial-mandibular movements for a subject with congenital spasticity without (upper panel) and with (lower panel) a bite-block.

shown in Figure 2-3, a logical step would be improvement of voluntary jaw control. Even helping this patient to position the jaw at a neutral height would be an improvement, because such a position would allow for more regular, smooth movement of other articulators, as was observed with the jaw fixed. These observations should not be interpreted as a suggestion that this dysarthric subject will ever regain control of the speech mechanism in a "normal" manner (e.g., conscious concentration upon careful positioning of the jaw may always be necessary) or as an argument for exclusive or primary use of nonspeech activities in therapy.

These interpretations have interesting implications for other forms of rehabilitation as well. For example, some treatments used in cerebral palsy have emphasized the facilitation of chewing and swallowing as a means for improving speech function. Despite the considerable zeal with which these programs are sometimes pursued, there is little direct evidence to support their value for speech improvement. The apparent difference in neural substrate for control of vegetative orofacial function and control of speech and nonspeech voluntary behavior argues against the utility of these therapies for speech. This argument appears to be supported by the recent observations of Love, Hagerman, and Taimi (1980), who found no consistent relation between severity of speech impairment in 60 children with cerebral palsy and the presence of dysphagia. Love and colleagues likewise reported the absence of a correlation between aberrations in oromotor reflexes and severity of speech impairment. This latter finding is consistent with interpretations suggesting that brainstem-mediated reflexes, posited earlier to be involved in speech motor control (McLean, Folkins, and Larson, 1979; Netsell and Abbs, 1975, 1977), subserve vegetative and protective functions; these brainstem reflex pathways appear to be largely inactive during the execution of normal speech production (Abbs and Cole, 1982; Abbs and Gracco, 1984; Gracco and Abbs, 1982). In particular, these observations emphasize the more direct role of cerebellar and cortical pathways in the normal speech motor control process, an interpretation that is consistent with that of Evarts (1981, 1982), as noted previously.

While these considerations offer a supporting basis for assessment and treatment of dysarthria via nonspeech voluntary control tasks, the details of this approach need to be considered in light of current "state-of-the-art" assessment procedures and their underlying neurophysiologic rationale. Regarding apraxia of speech, instrumental analyses of voluntary control of nonspeech behaviors in this population have not been conducted, to the knowledge of the authors of this chapter. Given the controversy surrounding this disorder, such analyses appear critical.

THEORETICAL EVALUATION
OF CURRENT ASSESSMENT
AND TREATMENT PROCEDURES

The treatment of dysarthria has increasingly involved emphasis upon more focused physical intervention, including biofeedback, palatal lifts, posturing, and abdominal binding (cf. Hixon, 1975; Netsell and Daniel, 1979; Rosenbek and LaPointe, 1978; Rubow, 1981; Rubow and Netsell, 1979). These physically oriented treatments, while often experimental, can be contrasted to earlier, more global approaches, in that optimal success may require detailed assessment of information concerning each patient's speech mechanism pathophysiology (Netsell and Daniel, 1979). To be more specific, it may not be optimal to utilize relaxation biofeedback to reduce muscle tone if the nature, degree, and distribution of that increased tone and its causal relation to speech performance deficits are not documented. Indeed, it is obvious that the long-term advancement of treatment intervention in both dysarthria and apraxia of speech depends as much upon the quality of the assessment in revealing the motor pathophysiology as upon the cleverness of the techniques themselves. Unfortunately, the effectiveness of current clinical assessment procedures in determining actual neuropathophysiology has not been evaluated systematically. Indeed, many assessment procedures for dysarthria are idiosyncratic to particular clinicians, making evaluation of their effectiveness difficult. To avoid imposing our own idiosyncracies, we will focus on assessment techniques that have been based upon published data.

As noted recently (cf. Abbs et al., 1983), assessment procedures, as they are advocated for use in many clinical settings, involve several serial steps if the diagnostician's purpose is to localize the lesion and to specify the apparent speech system neuropathophysiology. Initially, auditory-perceptual evaluation of the dysarthric speech is made, with attempts via speech task manipulations, to identify the nature of impairments in the major components of the speech production system (i.e., respiratory, phonatory, articulatory). This evaluation is augmented by a more or less standard oral-peripheral examination. Second, on the basis of formal or informal auditory-perceptual classification procedures (e.g., Darley, Aronson, and Brown, 1969a, 1969b, 1975) and knowledge of the parallel neurologic findings, differential categorization of the apparent neurologic syndrome is often considered. Many speech pathologists are extremely skilled at identifying certain disease clusters via auditory-perceptual analyses. Identification of the neurologic syndrome offers some insight into potential pathophysiology. However, despite the appeal of this step, inferences as to the "associated" movement and muscle contraction impairment manifestations in the speech production system are difficult. These inferences are commonly based on concurrent neurologic observations of the limb motor system and on classic, stereotypic descriptions of the syndrome-associated limb pathophysiology as provided in the limb movement disorders literature. For example, if the differential diagnosis yields the identification of hypokinetic dysarthria (for example, in Parkinson's disease), it is inferred (or assumed) that the speech motor impairment is a manifestation of rigidity, hypokinesia or bradykinesia, resting tremor, or a combination of these features in the muscles and movements of the speech production system. This pathophysiologic profile is, of course, a classic neurologic description of motor disorder signs in the limbs (Delong and Georgopoulos, 1981; Marsden, 1982). Aside from the difficulties with auditory-perceptual analyses of motor equivalence compensation discussed earlier, this assessment approach is based on two fundamental and related assumptions. The first assumption is that limb pathophysiology provides a valid basis for making inferences regarding associated speech motor problems. That is, there is an explicit assertion that the neuropathophysiology of movement disorders is manifest uniformly across limb and speech motor subsystems. This leads to a second assumption that the motor subsystems of the speech production system similarly are impaired uniformly as a result of a particular suprabulbar or supraspinal injury. In other words, the lips, tongue, jaw, larynx, pharynx, velopharynx, and respiratory system will show similar patterns of motor deficit. It is apparent that the validity of these two assumptions determines the degree to which these particular assessment procedures provide directions for treatment of the speech system pathophysiology.

These issues are perhaps most important if one considers the physiologic perspective of Hardy (1967) and the multicomponent representation of the speech production system that Netsell (1979) proposed as a guiding framework for physiologic assessment and treatment of motor speech disorders. As noted, this multicomponent orientation evolved from the argument that assessment of different speech motor subsystems is necessary to develop an optimal program of component-focused rehabilitation. This approach is particularly appealing in evaluating potential lower motoneuron disorders where differences in subsystem impairments might be present because of selective damage in some cranial nerves and not others. At issue, however, is whether it is necessary to conduct multiple subsystem assessment in dysarthrias of suprabulbar origin. While many experienced speech pathologists know the answer to this question, there is considerable value in offering a more detailed analysis with specific hypotheses. Hypothetically, if suprabulbar lesions uniformly impair all the motor subsystems of speech production system, evaluation of only one speech motor subsystem may be necessary. It could be possible to evaluate the control impairments in the most accessible speech motor subsystems (e.g., the lips) and infer the control impairments in the jaw, tongue, larynx, velum, and respiratory structures. However, if a suprabulbar lesion results in a nonuniform control impairment across the speech motor subsystems, determinations of speech motor impairment cannot be made from observations of a single motor subcomponent. Similarly, it would be difficult to make parallel inferences from limb motor impairments, as classically defined, to presumed pathophysiology in the orofacial system (cf. Darley et al., 1975). From the standpoint of motor neurophysiology (in determining the general validity of either the multiple speech component or the auditory-perceptual inferential assessment approaches), the question is whether the suprabulbar structures provide a uniform function in control of the body's motor subsystems. In short, *is the movement control required by the CNS uniform in nature for the limbs, abdomen, rib cage, larynx, pharynx, jaw, tongue and lips?* If the answer to the question is negative and the control requirements are substantially different, then damage at suprabulbar levels should yield nonuniform impairments among cranial and spinal motor subsystems.

There are several ways to approach these issues, the major avenues being analytic and empirical. To illustrate the value of a motor control approach as advocated previously, we should like to review the analytic considerations (i.e., examination of underlying limb and speech production subsystem motor neurophysiology), and, in parallel, note some recent physiologic observations of speech motor subsystem dysfunctions in subjects with "pure" suprabulbar impairments. A priori, the analytic approach offered by *systems physiology* is useful in evaluating the potential central nervous system control of different speech and spinal motor subsystems (cf. Milhorn, 1966; Partridge, 1976; Robinson, 1981a; Talbot and Gessner, 1973). This systems approach analysis requires that the major functional subsystem properties be identified and evaluated. As such, this evaluation, based upon current knowledge of motor physiology, yields the minimal subset of critical motor subsystem characteristics that must be considered for central nervous system control (cf. Muller, Abbs, and Kennedy, 1981). If these critical properties are functionally similar for different motor subsystems, we have reason to argue for CNS control uniformity. In addition to addressing the issue of speech-motor-subsystem-differential control and impairment, these considerations offer numerous testable hypotheses for focused research in speech motor disorders. For example, it is not very satisfying to simply acknowledge differential impairment. Rational therapy will flourish if we know, in pathophysiologic terms, why certain systems are differentially impaired.

The major components of a typical systems physiology–based neuromuscular model that are known to influence control can be readily identified (cf. Houk and Henneman, 1967; Houk and Rymer, 1981; Rack, 1981). These components include *system movement characteristics* (acceleration, velocity, and range of movement); *system biomechanics* (multimuscle geometry, muscle force generation characteristics, and passive mechanics including inertial, elastic, and viscous properties); *efferent activation of the muscles* (such as motoneuron innervation ratio, muscle fiber mechanical properties, and histochemical properties); *sensory innervation* (density and presence of muscle spindles, tendon organs, joint receptors, and cutaneous or mucosal mechanoreceptors); and *the pattern of efferent and afferent influences on the lower motoneuron pool*, including the distribution and nature of peripheral afferent influences, reciprocal or recurrent inhibition processes, and inputs from descending cortical pathways. These system physiology properties are of major significance in discerning how particular motor systems are controlled by the nervous system, as is reflected in a substantial body of evidence from experimental and mathematical analyses of motor systems in animals and human beings (cf. Houk, 1972; Houk and Rymer, 1981; Neilson, Andrews, Guitar, and Quinn, 1979; Rack, 1981; Robinson, 1981b).

On the basis of a neuromuscular subsystem evaluation of the properties of speech and limb motor subsystems, it is apparent that there are several critical physiologic and neurophysiologic differences. An illustration of the basis for this conclusion is the neuromuscular system profiles for a few speech and upper limb motor subsystems. These differences are evident even at the most peripheral level in the movement and biomechanical characteristics of these subsystems. The biomechanical properties of motor systems dictate the muscle contraction patterns (and hence CNS control signals) required to produce certain patterns of movement (cf. Abbs and Eilenberg, 1976; Houk, 1972; Houk and Henneman, 1967). For example, mass (inertial) properties impose an undeniable newtonian requirement upon the force necessary to movement up to a certain velocity. Likewise, "fluid friction" (viscosity) found in most biologic tissue requires proportional increases in muscle force as greater movement velocities are necessary. Thus, while slow movements of two motor subsystems can be activated in a comparable manner (with respect to the muscle contraction–CNS control signals), differences in acceleration or velocity for one system will require major control signal reorganization, depending upon their relative magnitudes of inherent inertia and viscosity (cf. Abbs and Muller, 1980; Pedotti, Krishnan, and Stark, 1978). From these data, one could predict with some confidence that the motor reorganization for changes in speech rate would require different processes for each speech motor subsystem, with further implications for the neurologically impaired. In relation to biomechanical comparisons of the lips, jaw, and upper limbs, we know that the lips do not have a significant inertial (mass) component, while these other movement systems require inclusion of inertia in their biomechanical profile (Abbs and Muller, 1980). It may be significant that the movements of the lips are generally more rapid than those of these other structures. Indeed, for slower speech movements, the lips can be controlled in a manner that is relatively more direct than comparable motor systems with significant inertial properties. Perhaps with certain forms of nervous system damage, control of lip movements would be less impaired than movements of other motor subsystems.

The potential influence of these movement and biomechanical characteristics upon control requirements is apparent when one considers the control of eye movements where different central nervous system mechanisms have been determined for rapid movements (saccadic), slow movements (smooth pursuit), and static positioning (fixation). That is, within the ocular motor system, there are documented neuroanatomic differences in the control network that vary as a function of movement demands (Robinson, 1981b). These different eye movements are selectively impaired by lesions of the nervous system (Phillips and Porter, 1977). On the basis of clinical observations, movement-dependent neural control differences have also been suggested by Kornhuber (1975), who proposed that postural movements are highly dependent upon the basal ganglia, while fast, "ballistic" movements are more dependent upon the cerebellar circuits. Obviously, if Kornhuber's distinction is useful, basal ganglia lesions should cause differential impairment among the various speech or limb motor subsystems, depending upon whether their movements are slow or fast.

As noted previously, recent investigations in both in limb and speech motor control document the moment-to-moment contributions of ascending afferent signals, operating at all levels of the motor programming process. Additionally, afferent control aberrations have played a prominent role in many theoretic models of movement disorders. Thus, in this context of potential control differences, it is useful to compare the nature of sensory innervation among motor subsystems. While the jaw and upper limbs have muscle spindle, joint, and tendon receptors (Harrison and Corbin, 1942;

Kubota, Masegi, and Osani, 1974; Lund, Richmond, Touloumis, Patry, and Lamarre, 1978), the lips have none of them (Folkins and Larson, 1978; Lovell, Sutton, and Lindeman, 1977), and the tongue has only muscle spindles (Bowman, 1968; Cooper, 1953; Fitzgerald and Sachithanandan, 1979). The larynx, like the jaw, apparently has each of these receptors (Baken, 1971; Larson, Sutton, and Lindeman, 1974; Lucas Keene, 1961). Clearly, if we assume, on the basis of current evidence, a role for these afferent systems in the control of movement, their differential distribution across motor subsystems indicates parallel differences in the required CNS control signals (cf. Houk and Rymer, 1981; Muller et al., 1981). Regarding motor impairments, it might be hypothesized that the hypertonus associated with spasticity would be greatest in motor subsystems where spindle afferents are abundant (cf. Landau, 1980).

Yet another important factor in the control required of the CNS is the nature of the neural influences (peripheral, central, and local) impinging upon the lower motoneuron pool. By definition, these influences must determine the final pattern of motoneuron signals to the muscle. Additionally, several prominent notions concerning pathophysiology implicate aberrant integration of influences impinging on these lower motoneurons. With regard to afferent influences on motoneurons, it is notable that while spindles in the jaw and upper limbs make monosynaptic connections, spindle afferents from the larynx and tongue are not so configured (Bowman and Combs, 1968; Bratzlavsky and vander Eecken, 1974; Neilson et al., 1979). For example, labial and lingual mechanoreceptor influences on motoneurons are known to be polysynaptic. However, it appears doubtful that lingual muscle spindles have any direct autogenic influence on the lingual motoneurons. Further, while spindle primary (IA) afferents in the limbs make connections to all motoneurons in a muscle, in the jaw, spindles appear to make connections only to smaller motoneurons (Appenteng, O'Donovan, Somjen, Stephens, and Taylor, 1978).

The nervous system control implications of these subsystem-dependent, afferent influences upon the lower motoneuron pool appear particularly significant, especially with regard to such phenomena as the size principle of motoneuron recruitment (cf. Burke, 1981; Henneman, Somjen, and Carpenter, 1965). The differential influences of spindle feedback on jaw motoneurons may influence their recruitment order. Inasmuch as the lips do not have spindles influencing the lower motoneuron pool, these muscles also are likely to show differences in motoneuron recruitment patterns in comparison to the limbs and jaw. A number of reports suggest motor neuropathologies have associated aberrations in motoneuron recruitment patterns (Milner-Brown, Stein, Lee, and Brown, 1980; Petajan, Jarcho, and Thurman, 1969). Finally, while patterns of recurrent and reciprocal inhibition are manifest for the upper limbs via lower motoneuron interactions with collaterals to inhibitory interneurons and spindle afferents, parallel processes do not appear to be operating for the cranial nerves. Rather, it appears that control of these important inhibitory patterns is regulated more centrally in the orofacial system (Dubner et al., 1978; Penders and Delwaide, 1973; Shahani and Young, 1973). Of major importance may be the potentially related fact that in primates (including human beings) motoneurons of the lips, jaw, tongue, and respiratory muscles receive monosynaptic inputs from corticomotor sites (Kuypers, 1958; Watson, 1973), while the motoneurons of the trunk and upper and lower limbs (independent of the digits) do not (Carpenter, 1976).

These neurophysiologic and neuroanatomic differences are almost irrefutable evidence that the central nervous system (CNS) does not control the limbs or the individual speech motor subsystems in the same manner. Indeed, a differential neuromuscular substrate appears to be the rule rather than the exception; the nature and size of motor-sensory and sensorimotor cortical representations make this conclusion painfully obvious. The inescapable prediction from these considerations, based upon specific and available evidence in the motor neurophysiology literature, is that damage to the CNS at a suprabulbar or supraspinal level will result in motor control impairments that are different among the speech production subsystems and the limbs. This conclusion is supported indirectly by even a casual perusal of the clinical neurophysiology literature. That is, hypogamma and hypergamma motor drive to muscle spindles, loss or aberrations in recurrent inhibition, and selective impairment of influences upon motoneuron pool recruitment patterns have all enjoyed some popularity as partial pathogenic explanations for spasticity, rigidity, tremor, ataxia, hypotonia, dysmetria, and asthenia. If some of these explanations are even partially correct, and because the implicated physiologic processes (e.g., presence of spindles, operation of recurrent inhibition) differ from one motor subsystem to another, then the neuropathophysiology must differ as well. This hypothesis has some support in observations of differential muscle contraction impairments between the upper and lower limbs (e.g., degrees of spasticity, rigidity, and tremor).

By way of direct support, several recent physiologic observations in parkinsonian ataxic, and spastic dysarthric patients indicate that such differential impairment among the motor subsystems of the speech production mechanism is the rule rather than the exception (Abbs et al., 1983; Barlow and Abbs, 1982; Hunker et al., 1982).

The implications of this ubiquitous nonuniformity of speech motor subsystem impairments are several. Initially, because global measures of the speech motor system may not in general permit one to discern impairments of individual articulators, determination of speech motor subsystem pathophysiology is enhanced by use of direct observations using voluntary, nonspeech tasks. In this manner, it may be possible to identify those speech motor subsystems manifesting the greatest degree of impairment and to focus treatment for maximum effectiveness. Improvements in speech motor function could possibly be enhanced by initial emphasis upon those subsystems that are either most severely impaired or allow for the most direct and effective intervention. This focused approach is thus contrasted to conventional, more globally oriented treatments. With these global treatments, it is assumed (or hoped) that if the dysarthric talker is given an overall behavioral target, inherent compensatory processes that are indiscernible to the therapist will allow for achievement of that objective. It may be, however, that optimal therapy must be focused in such a manner as to aid in those compensatory strategies. Perhaps without direct focus on the impairments in specific subsystems, the necessary compensatory adjustments may be indiscernible to the dysarthric talker as well. A particularly useful example of the importance of multimotor system evaluation offered by Abbs and colleagues (1983) was that of an adult with congenital spastic dysarthria. This person's condition was evaluated by a neurologist and a speech pathologist, both of whom observed the classic signs of spasticity and spastic dysarthria. Given this diagnosis, a uniform pattern of motor control impairment across the speech motor subsystems might be predicted. However, what was revealed from instrumental observation of the lip, tongue, and jaw control for nonspeech tasks was substantial weakness in the lips and tongue; control instability was present only in the jaw. Given this observation, it is likely that optimal treatment would involve some attempts at increasing strength in the lips and tongue, but a very different approach is necessary for improving jaw control. If a global strategy (e.g., general relaxation or positioning) had been used, these treatments might have been ineffective for the labial and lingual weakness that had gone undetected by the conventional speech or neurologic assessments. What is unfortunate about the phenomenon of differential speech motor subsystem impairments is that it has not been recognized and exploited earlier; the supporting data, the underlying motor control rationale, and the technology utilized have been available for over 20 years from work in motor neurophysiology and systems bioengineering.

CONCLUSION AND SUMMARY

While the foregoing discussions have dealt with some apparently important issues in the assessment and treatment of speech neuropathologies, these considerations represent only the tip of the proverbial iceberg. There are numerous examples of similarly significant questions that are addressed by current work in neurophysiology and motor disorders; for example, it was not possible, given the scope of this discussion, to also discuss (1) the demonstration that normal and disordered *cognitive* processes are a significant factor in motor programming and control (cf. Abbs and Kennedy, 1982; Marsden, 1982); (2) potential neurophysiologic mechanisms of compensatory patterns in individuals with motor disorders (Grimm and Nashner, 1978); (3) predictions of lesion sites in particular dysarthric populations and subpopulations based upon recent somatotopic investigations of orofacial and laryngeal representation in the basal ganglia, cerebellum, and cerebral cortex; (4) data-based definitions of movement and muscle contraction aberrations in patients with Parkinson's disease, congenital and acquired spasticity, or cerebellar impairment that replace and refine qualitative, semantically ambiguous terms such as akinesia, asthenia, and spasticity; or (5) a neurophysiologic rationale and specific methodology for the meaningful assessment of sensorimotor integrity as a potential factor in many speech motor neuropathologies. However, what is apparent from the issues discussed and this fundamental perspective is that some of the arguments occupying the energy of clinical scientists working on the speech neuropathologies become nonissues if all the available data are incorporated. From the standpoint of scientific integrity and underlying humanitarian objectives, speech neuropathologists cannot afford to be generalists, and hence they miss the substantial advances that have been made in the last ten years in the understanding of motor control and disorders thereof. Our clinical and research activities in this area must reflect the most relevant and recent information that the neurosciences have to offer. This wealth of information provides the basis from which we can further choose and refine those measures that provide the best insights into nervous system function and dysfunction. Professionally, adopting this approach may be critical, especially as new developments in areas such as clinical neurophysiology offer increasingly focused measures to discern specific aspects of nervous system function and dysfunction. That is, one danger of continuing traditional approaches (using borrowed measures that may yield ambiguous, albeit conventional data) is that the neurologist and physiologist will develop techniques for assessment of speech motor system function and dysfunction without the participation of individuals with primary education in the speech neuropathologies. Some work in this area is already under way, especially in Europe, where medically educated professionals conduct motor-sensory evaluations of the orofacial system in the neurologically impaired (cf. Bennett and Jannetta, 1980; Bratzlavsky, 1976; Dengler and Struppler, 1981; Schonle, 1982; Shahani and Young, 1973; Thumfart, 1981).

REFERENCES

Abbs, J. H. (1979). Speech motor equivalence: A need for a multilevel control model. In E. Fischer-Jorgenson, J. Rishcel, and N. Thorsen (Eds.), *Proceedings of the Ninth International Congress of Phonetics* (pp. 318–324). Denmark: Institute of Phonetics.

Abbs, J. H., and Cole, K. J. (1982). Consideration of bulbar and suprabulbar afferent influences upon speech motor coordination and programming. In S. Grillner, B. Lindblom, J. Lubker, and A. Persson (Eds.), *Speech motor control* (pp. 159–186). New York: Pergamon Press.

Abbs, J. H., and Eilenberg, G. R. (1976). Peripheral mechanisms of speech motor control. In N. J. Lass (Ed.), *Contemporary issues in experimental phonetics* (pp. 139–168). New York: Academic Press.

Abbs, J. H., and Gracco, V. L. (1982). Motor control of multi-movement behaviors. Orofacial muscle responses to load perturbations of the lips during speech. *Society for Neuroscience, 8,* 282 (Abstract).

Abbs, J. H., and Gracco, V. L. (1984). Control of complex motor gestures: Orofacial muscle responses to load perturbations of the lip during speech. *Journal of Neurophysiology, 51*(4), 705–723.

Abbs, J. H., Hunker, C. J., and Barlow, S. M. (1983). Differential speech motor subsystem impairments in subjects with suprabulbar lesions: Neurophysiological framework and supporting data. In W. Berry (Ed.), *Clinical dysarthria* (pp. 21–56). San Diego: College-Hill Press.

Abbs, J. H., and Kennedy, J. G. (1982). Neurophysiological processes of speech movement control. In N. J. Lass, L. V. McReynolds, J. L. Northern, and D. E. Yoder (Eds.), *Speech, language and hearing* (pp. 84–108). Philadelphia: W. B. Saunders.

Abbs, J. H., and Muller, E. M. (1980). *Neurophysiological and biomechanical factors in articulatory movement.* Paper presented at the Conference on the Production of Speech, Austin, Texas.

Abbs, J. H., Sutton, D., Larson, C., and Eilenberg, G. R. (1973). *Neuromuscular mechanisms underlying speech production (Program Project NINCDS NS11780).* Seattle: University of Washington.

Alexander, R. M. (1981). Biomechanics of skeleton and tendons. In V. B. Brooks (Ed.), *Handbook of physiology, Section 1 (Vol. II: Motor control, Part 1)* (pp. 17–42). Bethesda, MD: American Physiological Society.

Appenteng, K., O'Donovan, M. J., Somjen, G., Stephens, J. A., and Taylor, A. (1978.) The projection of jaw elevator muscle spindle afferents to fifth nerve motoneurons in the cat. *Journal of Physiology, 279,* 409–423.

Baken, R. J. (1971). Neuromuscular spindles in the intrinsic muscles of the human larynx. *Folia Phoniatrica, 23,* 204–210.

Barlow, S. M., and Abbs, J. H. (1982). Impairment control of orofacial muscle force in congenital spastics. *Society for Neuroscience, 8* (Part 2), 953 (Abstract).

Barlow, S. M., and Abbs, J. H. (1984). Orofacial fine motor control impairments in congenital spastics: Evidence against muscle spindle-related performance deficits. *Neurology, 34,* 145–150.

Bennett, M. H., and Jannetta, P. H. (1980). Trigeminal evoked potentials in humans. *EEG Clinical Neurophysiology, 48,* 517–526.

Bernstein, N. (1967). *The co-ordination and regulation of movements.* Oxford: Pergamon Press.

Bowman, J. P. (1968). Muscle spindles in the intrinsic and extrinsic muscles of the Rhesus monkey's *(Macaca mulatta)* tongue. *Anatomical Record, 161,* 483–488.

Bowman, J. P., and Combs, C. M. (1968). Discharge patterns of lingual spindle afferent fibers in the hypoglossal nerve of the Rhesus monkey. *Experimental Neurology, 21,* 105–119.

Bratzlavsky, M. (1976). The connections between muscle afferents and motoneurons of the muscles of mastication. In D. J. Anderson and B. Matthews (Eds.), *Mastication* (pp. 147–151). Bristol: Wright.

Bratzlavsky, M., and vander Eecken, H. (1974). Afferent influences on human genioglossus muscle. *Journal of Neurology, 207,* 19–25.

Brooks, V. B. (1981). *Handbook of physiology, Section 1 (Vols. I and II: Motor control, Parts 1 and 2).* Bethesda, MD: American Physiological Society.

Burke, R. E. (1981). Motor units: anatomy, physiology and functional organization. In V. B. Brooks (Ed.), *Handbook of physiology, Section 1 (Vol. II: Motor control, Part 1)* (pp. 345–422). Bethesda, MD: American Physiological Society.

Carpenter, M. B. (1976). *Human neuroanatomy.* Baltimore: Williams & Wilkins.

Cooper, S. (1953). Muscle spindles in the intrinsic muscles of the human tongue. *Journal of Physiology, 122,* 193–202.

Darley, F. L., Aronson, A. E., and Brown, J. R. (1969a). Differential diagnostic patterns of dysarthria. *Journal of Speech and Hearing Research, 12,* 246–269.

Darley, F. L., Aronson, A. E., and Brown, J. R. (1969b). Cluster of deviant speech dimensions in the dysarthrias. *Journal of Speech and Hearing Research, 12,* 462–496.

Darley, F. L., Aronson, A. E., and Brown, J. R. (1975). *Motor speech disorders.* Philadelphia: W. B. Saunders.

DeLong, M., and Georgopoulos, A. P. (1981). Motor functions of the basal ganglia. In V. B. Brooks (Ed.), *Handbook of physiology, Section 1 (Vol. II: Motor control, Part 2)* (pp. 1017–1062). Bethesda, MD: American Physiological Society.

Dengler, R., and Struppler, A. (1981). Neurophysiological diagnosis of trigeminal nerve function. In M. Sammii and P. Jannetta (Eds.), *The cranial nerves* (pp. 302–311). Berlin: Springer-Verlag.

Denny-Brown, D. (1960). Motor mechanisms—Introduction: The general principles of motor integration. In H. W. Magoun (Ed.), *Handbook of physiology, Section 1* (pp. 781–796). Washington, DC: American Physiological Society.

Denny-Brown, D. (1980). Preface: Historical aspects of the relation of spasticity to movement. In R. G. Feldman, R. R. Young, and W. P. Koella (Eds.), *Spasticity: Disordered motor control* (pp. 1-16). Chicago: Year Book Medical Publishers.

Desmedt, J. E. (Ed.) (1973-1982). *Progress in clinical neurophysiology (10 vols.)*. Basel: S. Karger.

Dubner, R., Sessle, B. J., and Storey, A. T. (1978). *The neural basis of oral and facial function.* New York: Plenum.

Duncan, G. W., Shahani, B. T., and Young, R. R. (1976). An evaluation of baclofen treatment for certain symptoms in patients with spinal cord lesions. A double cross-over study. *Neurology, 26,* 441-446.

Evarts, E. V. (1981). Role of motor cortex in voluntary movements in primates. In V. B. Brooks (Ed.), *Handbook of physiology, Section 1 (Vol. II: Motor control, Part 2)* (pp. 1083-1120). Bethesda, MD: American Physiological Society.

Evarts, E. V. (1982). Analogies between central motor programs for speech and limb movements. In S. Grillner, B. Lindblom, J. Lubker, and A. Persson (Eds.), *Speech motor control* (pp. 19-42). London: Pergamon Press.

Fitzgerald, M. J. T., and Sachithanandan, S. R. (1979). The structure and source of lingual proprioceptors in the monkey. *Journal of Anatomy, 128*(3), 523-552.

Folkins, J. W., and Abbs, J. H. (1975). Lip and jaw motor control during speech: Responses to resistive loading of the jaw. *Journal of Speech and Hearing Research, 18,* 207-220.

Folkins, J. W., and Abbs, J. H. (1976). Additional observations on responses to resistive loading of the jaw. *Journal of Speech and Hearing Research, 19,* 820-821.

Folkins, J. W., and Larson, C. R. (1978). In search of a tonic vibration reflex in the human lip. *Brain Research, 151,* 409-412.

Fujimura, O. (1981). Temporal organization of articulatory movements as a multi-dimensional phrasal structure. *Phonetica, 38,* 66-83.

Gentil, M., Gracco, V. L., and Abbs, J. H. (1983). Multiple muscle contributions to labial closure during speech: Evidence for inter-muscle motor equivalence. *Proceedings of the 11th International Congress of Acoustics,* pp. 11-14 (Abstract).

Gracco, V. L., and Abbs, J. H. (1982). Temporal response characteristics of the perioral system to load perturbations. *Society for Neuroscience, 8,* (Part 2), 282 (Abstract).

Gracco, V. L., and Muller, E. M. (1981, November). *Analysis of supraglottal air pressure variations in spastic dysarthria.* Paper presented at the American Speech, Language, and Hearing Association, Los Angeles.

Granit, R. (1977). *The purposive brain.* Cambridge, MA: MIT Press.

Grimm, R. J., and Nashner, L. M. (1978). Long loop dyscontrol. In J. E. Desmedt (Ed.), *Cerebral motor control in man: Long loop mechanisms* (Vol. 4) (pp. 70-84). Basel: S. Karger.

Hardy, J. C. (1967). Suggestions for physiological research in dysarthria. *Cortex, 3,* 128-156.

Hardy, J. C. (1970). Development of neuromuscular systems underlying speech production. *ASHA Reports: Speech and the Dentofacial Complex: The State of the Art, Proceedings of the Workshop, 5,* 49-68.

Harrison, F., and Corbin, K. B. (1942). The central pathway for the jaw-jerk. *American Journal of Physiology, 135,* 439-445.

Hebb, D. O. (1949). *The organization of behavior.* New York: John Wiley and Sons.

Henneman, E., Somjen, G., and Carpenter, D. O. (1965). Excitability and inhibitability of motoneurons of different sizes. *Journal of Neurophysiology, 28,* 599-620.

Hixon, T. J. (1963). *Restricted motility of the speech articulators in cerebral palsy.* Unpublished master's thesis, University of Iowa.

Hixon, T. J. (1975). *Respiratory-laryngeal evaluation*. Paper presented at the Veterans Administration Workshop on Motor Speech Disorders, Madison, Wisconsin.

Hixon, T. J., and Hardy, J. C. (1964). Restricted mobility of the speech articulators in cerebral palsy. *Journal of Speech and Hearing Disorders, 29,* 293-306.

Hoffman, D. S., and Luschei, E. S. (1980). Responses of monkey precentral cortical cells during a controlled jaw bite task. *Journal of Neurophysiology, 44,* 333-348.

Houk, J. C. (1972). On the significance of various command signals during voluntary control. *Brain Research, 40,* 49-53.

Houk, J. C., and Henneman, E. (1967). The feedback control of skeletal muscles. *Brain Research, 5,* 433-451.

Houk, J. C. and Rymer, W. Z. (1981). Neural control of muscle length and tension. In V. B. Brooks (Ed.), *Handbook of physiology, Section 1 (Vol. II: Motor control, Part 1)* (pp. 257-323). Bethesda, MD: American Physiological Society.

Hughes, O. M., and Abbs, J. H. (1976). Labial-mandibular coordination in the production of speech: Implications for the operation of motor equivalence. *Phonetica, 44,* 199-221.

Hunker, C. J., and Abbs, J. H. (1982). Respiratory movement control during speech: Evidence for motor equivalence. *Society for Neuroscience, 8* (Part 2), 946 (Abstract).

Hunker, C. J., and Abbs, J. H. (1984). Physiological analyses of parkinsonian tremors in the orofacial system. In M. R. McNeil, J. C. Rosenbek, and A. E. Aronson (Eds.), *The dysarthrias: Physiology-acoustics-perception-management* (pp. 69-100). San Diego: College-Hill Press.

Hunker, C. J., Abbs, J. H., and Barlow, S. M. (1982). The relationship between Parkinson rigidity and hypokinesia in the orofacial system: A quantitative analysis. *Neurology, 32*(7), 749-754.

Kornhuber, H. H. (1975). Cerebral cortex, cerebellum, and basal ganglia: An introduction to their motor function. In E. V. Evarts (Ed.), *Central processing of sensory input leading to motor output.* Cambridge, MA: MIT Press.

Kubota, K., Masegi, T., and Osani, K. (1974). Muscle spindle in masticatory muscle and its trigeminal mesencephalic nucleus. *Bulletin of the Tokyo Medical and Dental University* (Suppl. 21), 3-6.

Kuypers, H. G. J. M. (1958). Corticobulbar connections to the pons and lower brainstem in man: An anatomical study. *Brain, 81,* 364-388.

Lacquaniti, F., and Soechting, J. F. (1982). Coordination of arm and wrist motion during a reaching task. *Journal of Neuroscience, 2,* 399-408.

Ladefoged, P., DeClark, J., Lindau, M., and Papcun, G. (1972). An auditory-motor theory of speech production. *UCLA Working Papers in Phonetics, 22,* 48-75.

Lance, J. W. (1980). Pathophysiology of spasticity and clinical experience with baclofen. In R. G. Feldman, R. R. Young, and W. P. Koella (Eds.), *Spasticity: Disordered motor control* (pp. 185-203). Chicago: Year Book Medical Publishers.

Landau, W. M. (1974). Spasticity: The fable of a neurological demon and the emperor's new therapy. *Archives of Neurology, 31,* 217-219.

Landau, W. M. (1980). Spasticity: What is it? What is it not? In R. G. Feldman, R. R. Young, and W. P. Koella (Eds.), *Spasticity: Disordered motor control* (pp. 17-24). Chicago: Year Book Medical Publishers.

Larson, C. R., Sutton, D., and Lindeman, R. C. (1974). Muscle spindles in non-human primate laryngeal muscles. *Folia Primatologia, 22,* 315-325.

Lashley, K. S. (1930). Basic neural mechanisms in behavior. *Psychological Review, 37,* 1-24.

Lindau, M., Jacobson, L., and Ladefoged, P. (1972). The feature advanced tongue root. *UCLA Working Papers in Phonetics, 22.*

Lindblom, B. (1982). The interdisciplinary challenge of speech motor control. In S. Grillner, B. Lindblom, J. Lubker, and A. Persson (Eds.), *Speech motor control* (pp. 3-18). London: Pergamon Press.

Love, R. J., Hagerman, E. L., and Taimi, E. G. (1980). Speech performance, dysphagia and oral reflexes in cerebral palsy. *Journal of Speech and Hearing Disorders, 45*, 59-75.

Lovell, M., Sutton, D., and Lindeman, R. (1977). Muscle spindles in non-human primate extrinsic auricular muscles. *Anatomical Record, 189*, 519-524.

Lucas Keene, M. F. (1961). Muscle spindles in human laryngeal muscles. *Journal of Anatomy, 95*, 25-29.

Lund, J. P., Richmond, F. J. R., Touloumis, C., Patry, Y., and Lamarre, Y. (1978). The distribution of ganglia tendon organs and muscle spindles in the masseter and temporalis muscles of the cat. *Neuroscience, 3*, 259-270.

Marsden, C. D. (1982). The mysterious motor function of the basal ganglia. *Neurology, 32*, 514-539.

McClean, M. D., Folkins, J. W., and Larson, C. R. (1979). The role of the perioral reflex in lip motor control for speech. *Brain and Language, 7*, 42-61.

Milhorn, H. T. (1966). *The application of control theory to physiological systems*. Philadephia: W. B. Saunders.

Milner-Brown, H. S., Stein, R. B., Lee, R. G., and Brown, W. F. (1980). Motor unit recruitment in patients with neuromuscular disorders. In J. E. Desmedt (Ed.), *Motor unit types, recruitment and plasticity in health and disease (Progress in clinical neurophysiology, Vol. 9)* (pp. 305-318). Basel: S. Karger.

Morasso, P. (1981). Spatial control of arm movements. *Experimental Brain Research, 42*, 223-227.

Muller, E. M., Abbs, J. H., and Kennedy, J. G. (1981). Some system physiology considerations for vocal control. In M. Hirano and K. Stevens (Eds.), *Proceedings of the conference on vocal fold physiology* (pp. 209-227). Tokyo: University of Tokyo Press.

Muller, E. M., and Brown, W. S. (1980). Variations in the supraglottal air pressure waveform and their articulatory interpretation. In N. J. Lass (Ed.), *Speech and language: Advances in basic research and practice* (pp. 317-389). New York: Academic Press.

Murphy, M. W. (1966). *Speech physiology problems in athetoid and spastic quadriplegic children*. Unpublished master's thesis, University of Iowa.

Nashner, L. M., and Grimm, R. J. (1978). Analysis of multiloop dyscontrols in standing cerebellar patients. In J. E. Desmedt (Ed.), *Cerebral motor control in man: Long loop mechanisms* (Vol. 4) (pp. 300-319). Basel: S. Karger.

Neilson, P. D., Andrews, G., Guitar, B. E., and Quinn, P. T. (1979). Tonic stretch reflexes in lip, tongue and jaw muscles. *Brain Research, 178*, 311-327.

Netsell, R. (1971-1976). Physiological studies of the dysarthrias. *Final Progress Report— NINCDS Research Grant.*

Netsell, R., and Abbs, J. H. (1975, October). *The modulation of perioral reflex sensitivity during speech movements*. Paper presented at the Acoustical Society of America, San Francisco.

Netsell, R., and Abbs, J. H. (1977). Some possible uses of neuromotor speech disturbances in understanding the normal mechanism. In M. Sawashima and F. S. Cooper (Eds.), *Dynamic aspects of speech production* (pp. 369-392). Tokyo: University of Tokyo Press.

Netsell, R., and Daniel, B. (1979). Dysarthria in adults: Physiological approach to rehabilitation. *Archives of Physical Medicine and Rehabilitation, 60*, 502-508.

Partridge, L. (1976). A proposal for study of a static description of the motor control system. In M. Shahani (Ed.), *The motor system: Neurophysiological and muscle mechanics* (pp. 363-370). New York: Elsevier.

Partridge, L. D., and Benton, L. A. (1981). Muscle, the motor. In V. B. Brooks (Ed.), *Handbook of physiology, Section 1 (Vol. II: Motor control, Part 1)* (pp. 43–106). Bethesda, MD: American Physiological Society.

Pedotti, A., Krishnan, V. V., and Stark, L. (1978). Optimization of muscle force sequencing in human locomotion. *Mathematical Biosciences, 38*, 57–76.

Penders, C. A., and Delwaide, P. J. (1973). Physiological approach to the human blink relflex. In J. E. Desmedt (Ed.), *New developments in electromyography and clinical neurophysiology* (pp. 649–657). Basel: S. Karger.

Petajan, J. H., Jarcho, L. W., and Thurman, D. J. (1969). Motor unit control in Huntington's disease: a possible presymptomatic test. In J. Chase (Ed.), *Advances in neurology* (pp. 163–176). New York: Raven Press.

Phillips, C. G., and Porter, R. (1977). *Corticospinal neurones. Their role in movement.* London: Academic Press.

Rack, P. M. H. (1981). Limitations of somatosensory feedback in control of posture and movement. In V. B. Brooks (Ed.), *Handbook of physiology, Section 1 (Vol. II: Motor control, Part 1)* (pp. 229–256). Bethesda, MD: American Physiological Society.

Robinson, D. A. (1981a). The use of control systems analysis in neurophysiology of eye movements. *Annual Review of Neuroscience, 4*, 463–503.

Robinson, D. A. (1981b). Control of eye movements. In V. B. Brooks (Ed.), *Handbook of physiology, Section 1 (Vol. II: Motor control, Part 2)* (pp. 1275–1320). Bethesda, MD: American Physiological Society.

Rosenbek, J. C., and LaPointe, L. (1978). The dysarthrias: Description, diagnosis, and treatment. In D. F. Johns (Ed.), *Clinical management of neurogenic communicative disorders* (pp. 251–310). Boston: Little, Brown.

Rubow, R. T. (1981). Biofeedback in the treatment of speech disorders. *Biofeedback Society of America Task Force Reports.*

Rubow, R. T., and Netsell, R. (1979). EMG biofeedback rehabilitation in facial paralysis: Ten year follow-up of a case study. *Proceedings of the Tenth Annual Meeting of the Biofeedback Society of America,* San Diego, California.

Sahrman, S. A., and Norton, B. J. (1977). The relationship of voluntary movement to spasticity in the upper motor neuron syndrome. *Annals of Neurology, 2*, 460–465.

Schonle, P. W. (1982). Personal communication.

Shahani, B. T., and Young, R. R. (1973). Blink reflexes in orbicularis oculi. In J. E. Desmedt (Ed.), *New developments in electromyography and clinical neurophysiology* (pp. 641–648). Basel: S. Karger.

Smit, A. (1969). *Relationship of select physiological variables to speech defectiveness of athetoid and spastic cerebral palsied children.* Unpublished master's thesis, University of Iowa.

Smith, L. L. (1964). *Restricted motility of the speech articulators, lung function, amount of air expired per unit of speech and speech defectiveness in adults with Parkinson's disease.* Unpublished master's thesis, University of Iowa.

Stalberg, E., and Young, R. R. (1981). *Clinical neurophysiology.* Boston: Butterworths International Medical Reviews.

Stevens, K. N., and House, A. S. (1955). Development of a quantitative description of vowel articulation. *Journal of the Acoustical Society of America, 27*, 484–493.

Stevens, K. N., and House, A. S. (1961). An acoustical theory of vowel production and some of its implications. *Journal of Speech and Hearing Research, 4*, 303–320.

Sussman, H. M., MacNeilage, P. F., and Hanson, R. J. (1973). Labial and mandibular dynamics during the production of bilabial stop consonants. *Journal of Speech and Hearing Research, 16*, 385–396.

Talbot, S. A., and Gessner, U. (1973). *Systems physiology.* New York: John Wiley and Sons.

Thumfart, W. (1981). Endoscopic electroneurography and neurography. In M. Sammii and P. Jannetta (Eds.), *The cranial nerves* (pp. 597–606). Berlin: Springer-Verlag.

Watson, C. (1973). Functional deficits and the patterns of degeneration following lesions of the face motor cortex in the *Macaca mulatta. Anatomical Review, 175,* 465.

Wyke, B. (Ed.) (1974). *Ventilatory and phonatory control systems.* London: Oxford University Press.

Chapter 3

The Phonologic System: Problems of Second Language Acquisition

Walt Wolfram

Learning to speak a foreign language involves learning another phonologic system. While the acquisition of this second language system (L2) may be likened in some respects to learning the phonology of the first language (L1), there are obvious and important differences (Macken and Ferguson, 1981). In the acquisition of the native language phonologic system, certain natural and universal phonologic processes have to be overcome in learning the specific patterns of the adult language. In the acquisition of a foreign language as an adult, it is primarily the phonologic patterns of the first and native language that have to be overcome in learning the new system. Failure to overcome the L1 (i.e., native language) patterns of phonology in speaking the L2 (i.e., the target language) results in the classically defined "foreign accent." Technically, this is called language *interference* or *transfer*, referring to the fact that the patterns of the native language may be imposed on the target language.

The focus on language transfer in L2 phonologic acquisition is not intended to preclude other explanations. Certainly, some evidence suggests that other phenomena account for some adaptation of the L2 system as well (Tarone, 1976; Wode, 1977). For example, there may be a reactivation of the L1 developmental processes akin to those described in the recent emphasis on natural phonologic processes (Ingram, 1976; Stampe, 1973), or modifications that derive from particular L2 learning strategies (Wolfram, 1983). Nonetheless, the burden of explanation in adult L2 phonologic acquisition still rests on language transfer. This continued (and, in fact, renewed) emphasis on transfer in L2 phonology clearly contrasts with the trend in L2 syntax, where evidence over the past decade has emphasized the role of generalized learning strategies rather than language transfer (Burt and Kiparsky, 1972; Corder, 1981; Dulay and Burt, 1972).

In phonology, evidence (Oller, 1974; Sato, 1983) continues to point to the primary role of transfer for adult learners. Thus, a basic transfer model, with appropriate modifications, has weathered the challenge of empirically based L2 studies of the past decade. Given the state of the art, our goal is to present a coherent model that integrates current insights about variation and phonologic organization rather than simple recitation of recent research.

The range of transfer manifested by a given talker may vary, but in all cases we can expect the language codes to interact systematically. Speakers of a given native language background typically make similar kinds of "errors" when learning a foreign language, and this patterned behavior is the keynote to this discussion. We are dealing with systematic, patterned phonologic behavior that results from the normal interaction of two phonologic systems. While the resultant phonology may be quite different from the adult native speaker phonology, it can hardly be called a "disorder" in the traditional applications of this term. It is simply the normal result of imposing another phonologic system on one already established, and should be considered a kind of *interlanguage* norm. Nonetheless, this normal interlanguage behavior may lead to communication problems for talkers desiring to become more proficient in their phonology for various sociocultural reasons, so that it is a relevant topic for discussion here. In the following sections, we shall examine some aspects of phonologic organization in learning a second language, propose a model for understanding the acquisition of a second phonology, and finally discuss relevant pedagogic issues for language teachers, including diagnosis and remediation by speech-language pathologists.

The comparison of language systems related to foreign language learning has become a specialized field in its own right, often referred to as *contrastive linguistics.* Basic to this field is the comparison of structures in the native and target languages of the language learner in order to understand particular foreign language learner difficulties. While some aspects of contrastive linguistics have proved particularly troublesome on a theoretic and practical level (Wardhaugh, 1970), it is unarguable that the comparison of native and target language phonologies leads to considerable insight concerning the nature of learner problems. All levels of phonologic organization may be compared, including the underlying phonologic units, particular phonologic rules or processes, and surface phonemic contrasts. Traditionally, however, the emphasis has been on the interaction of systems on the more concrete levels of phonology—the surface phonemic contrasts. On the basis of a classic summary of inventories of phonemes and their allophones, Weinreich (1953) distinguished four different kinds of phonologic interaction and interference. These categories remain useful despite recent developments in redefining the basic units of a phonologic system.*

UNDERDIFFERENTIATION

This takes place when two or more contrastive sounds of the target language are treated as noncontrastive, because no phonologic contrast exists for these sounds in the native language. For example, Spanish does not contrast *s* and *z*; [z] is an allophone of [s]. English on the other hand, contrasts these sounds in items such as *sip* [sIp] and *zip* [sIp]. Thus, in learning English, a speaker of Spanish may not differentiate between the [s] and [z] contrast, possibly confusing items such as *sip* and *zip*, or *peace* and *peas*. Because underdifferentiation of this type can obviously lead to confusion among vocabulary items, it is considered one of the more serious types of phonologic interference. A similar problem of underdifferentiation might be faced by the English speaker learning an Asian language such as Hindi. In Hindi, the difference between aspirated and unaspirated stops is contrastive. English speakers who treat [p] and [pʰ], or [k] and [kʰ], as if they were part of the same contrastive unit (as they are in English) underdifferentiate the contrastive units of Hindi.

OVERDIFFERENTIATION

In overdifferentiation, contrasts from the native language are applied to the sounds of the target language, even though they are not required by the target language phonologic system. For example, an English speaker learning Spanish might consider [s] and [z] to be contrastive items in Spanish because they are contrastive in English. But as we noted, [s] and [z] are not contrastive sounds in Spanish, so that their conceptual differentiation is not necessary. Similarly, a Hindi speaker learning English might treat [p] and [pʰ] as if they were different contrastive units. Cases of overdifferentiation may not affect production in any significant way, but the learner's conception of contrastive units will differ from that of the native speaker. Understandably, overdifferentiation does not lead to the confusion among lexical items that underdifferentiation might. It is

---

*This section is adapted from Wolfram and Johnson (1982).

therefore not usually considered a problem in foreign language learning. Nonetheless, it must be recognized as one type of interaction between phonologic systems that affects the ways in which the units of the native language and the target language are conceptualized.

REINTERPRETATION OF DISTINCTIONS

In the reinterpretation of distinctions, the contrast of units in the target language is maintained, but on a basis different from that found in the native language. Thus, phonetic features that are redundant in the target language may be used as the basis for maintaining contrast by the native language speaker. Consider how a speaker of German learning English may utilize vowel length contrastively in a context where an English speaker may utilize vowel length redundantly. In both instances, the end result is the differentiation of items, but on a different basis. German uses phonetic differences in vowel length to distinguish items. The difference between [štat] "city" and [šta:t] "state," and [kan] "can" and [ka:n] "boat," is indicated by the length of the vowel. In English, however, length is typically much more predictable on the basis of the following environment. Vowels are lengthened before voiced segments ([bI:d] "bid"), and unlengthened before voiceless segments ([bIt] "bit").

Another difference between German and English phonology relates to the voicing of obstruents (i.e., stops and fricatives) in word-final position. In German, only voiceless obstruents are produced in this position, whereas in English both voiced and voiceless obstruents are found. Using the German word-final devoicing pattern, German speakers will often devoice the final voiced obstruents on English items such as *bead, pig,* and *buzz.* Despite the devoicing of the final obstruents, however, contrast may be maintained for German speakers confronted with these English items. The German speaker who devoices final obstruents may use the length of the preceding vowel rather than the voicing contrast to distinguish items, producing *bead* [bi:t] and *beat* [bit], *pig* [pI:k] and *pick* [pIk], *buzz* [bʌ:s] and *bus* [bʌs]. In an informal experiment conducted by the author, it was clearly indicated that native German speakers were cueing on the vowel length rather than final voicing to distinguish these items. Thus, we see that English redundant features may take on distinctive status for speakers from a different language background.

ACTUAL PHONE SUBSTITUTION

In phone substitution, the contrastive units of the native language and target language are comparable in terms of their contrastive status, but their phonetic production differs. For example, the German and French lateral *l* may be considered to be equivalent to English *l*, but the phonetic production may be different. German and French employ only the alveolar or "clear" [l], whereas English often produces an alveovelar lateral or "dark" [ɫ]. The difference in phonetic production may not lead to any particular confusion in terms of contrastive units, but the use of the English [ɫ] in speaking French or German will sound somewhat accented. Similarly, the exclusive use of [l] by French or German speakers using English will sound slightly accented in certain environments where English uses [ɫ].

PHONOTACTIC DIFFERENCES

We have just examined the interaction of the native and target languages only in terms of the basic inventory of units. But phonologic systems also are highly patterned in terms of the permissible sequences of sounds, referred to as *phonotactic patterning*. Thus, English has particular combinations of sounds in a linear string that may or may not be comparable to those found in other languages. Phonotactic differences are just as likely to lead to second language learning problems as are differences in the basic inventory of units.

There are several ways in which phonotactic differences may lead to problems for the second language learner. In some cases, the distribution patterns of segments within syllables may be different across language systems. Both English and Tagalog distinguish three nasals, [m], [n], and [ŋ], but English does not use [ŋ] in syllable-initial position, whereas Tagalog does. An English speaker confronted with items such as Tagalog [ŋaʔ] "really" and [ŋakŋa:k] "cry aloud" may therefore encounter difficulty producing the [ŋ] in these positions. This is a result not of a contrastive difference but of a difference in the distributional privileges within the syllable. Another difference in distribution between Tagalog and English is the occurrence of [h]. In Tagalog, [h] may occur in the syllable-final position, whereas in English it may not. Thus, Tagalog items such as [amah] "father" and [tu:boh] "tube" reveal a pattern not found in English. The native English speaker will tend to eliminate the final [h].

Major differences in phonotactics often concern sequences of segments of consonants or consonants and vowels. Syllable types and segment cluster types differ across phonologic systems, and these differences are often revealed in the kinds of problems found among second language learners. For example, Spanish does not permit syllable-initial sibilant + stop sequences, as in English *sp, st,* or *sk.* Thus, Spanish speakers impose the Spanish phonotactic system and produce these English clusters with a prothetic vowel ([ɛstʌdi] for *study* or [ɛskul] for *school*). In a parallel way, an English speaker learning German may be confronted with certain syllable-initial sequences not permissible in English. These include velar stops + nasals (German [knabə] "boy" and [gnadə] "mercy") and stops + fricatives ([psalm] "psalm" [pfʊnt] "pound"). Two possibilities exist here for imposing the English phonotactic structure. Speakers might use an epenthetic vowel to separate the nonpermissible English sequence ([kənabə]), or reduce the cluster by deleting one of the members ([nabə] or [fʊnt]). In both cases, the modification would result in a permissible English syllable type, but an unusual German pronunciation. Our examples might be expanded here, but the essential point remains the same: many second language learning problems may be attributable to differences in the sequencing of sounds rather than in the sound units themselves, and these differences must be taken into account along with differences in the inventory of units.

PHONOLOGIC PROCESSES

Much recent work in phonology (e.g., Ingram, 1976; Wolfram and Johnson, 1982) has recognized that language differences are susceptible to a number of different phonologic processes that alter the shape of units. Because of the natural basis for various processes, it is not surprising to see similar processes in two different language systems. There is, for example, a class of nasal prefixes in Swahili that is conditioned by the place of articulation of the following segment (*m-bari* "clan," *n-devu* "beard," *ŋ-guzo* "post"). This *assimilation* is similar to the form changes found in English (*impossible, indefinite, inconclusive*). But while recognizing certain similarities in the types of phonologic processes found in different systems on the basis of some universal principles, we must also observe significant differences in detail as we compare phonologic systems.

Many language systems may employ *neutralization* of one type or another, but the particular details of neutralization will vary greatly. Thus, the English talker shows extensive neutralization of vowels in unstressed syllables, so most English vowels can reduce to [ə]. Spanish, on the other hand, reveals little vowel neutralization of this type, maintaining contrasts in unstressed syllables as well as stressed ones. By the same token, standard English does not have the broadly applied German rule of final obstruent devoicing. Neutralization of contrasts in unstressed syllables, or devoicing in word-final position, may qualify as natural processes, but the particular details of these processes and the extent of their operation show considerable variation between systems. Such diversity is an important aspect of comparing systems in a contrastive analysis.

Similarly, languages commonly have *deletion* processes, but they may differ in details. Thus, French has a rule in which many word-final consonants are deleted when the following word begins with a consonant (e.g., [pəti garsɔ̃] "little boy") but not when followed by a vowel (e.g., [pətit ami] "little friend"). The application of this rule to English by a native French speaker might result in the deletion of consonants in similar contexts in English, so that the talker might produce [bɛ gem] (bed game) but [bɛt ɔfər] (bet offer). In this instance, the primary difference is the transfer of a process or rule from the native language to the target language rather than a difference in the basic inventory or phonotactic structure of the language. Thus, the comparison of processes or rules across language systems is another dimension of phonologic organization that has to be taken into account in examining the interaction of two language systems. The application of native language processes to a second language will potentially create still another kind of phonologic interference.

The consideration of phonologic processes in L2 acquisition is a point at which the transfer model is in need of some qualification. Some phonologic processes appear to have a natural, universal basis rather than a language specific one, so that they may have an explanation that is independent of language. For example, Wolfram (1983) shows that certain final consonant deletion processes are operative in the L2 English of L1 Vietnamese speakers despite the fact that the particular final consonants are present in both the L1 and L2 languages. In a study of syllable structure processes by Tarone (1976), it was found that 10 per cent to 47 per cent of all L2 phonologic errors could not be attributed to a transfer source. Given such evidence, Mulford and Hecht (1980) suggest that there is an interaction between transfer and natural universal processes. They further suggest that the relative roles of universally based processes and transfer processes from L1 differ according to the class of sounds involved. They offer the following continuum of relative effect:

Vowels   Liquids   Stops   Fricatives/Affricates

◄───►

Transfer   Developmental
processes   processes
predominate   predominate

Although such a continuum seems reasonable, it is still speculative, and in need of empirical justification. Furthermore, it seems much more applicable to children than adults. While adults certainly can reactivate L1 strategies to some extent in the L2 situation, current evidence (e.g., Oller, 1974; Sato, 1983) still points to the primary role of transfer.

VARIATION AND SECOND LANGUAGE LEARNING

At first glance, the phonology of a second language learner may appear to consist of a random set of language errors. While there is certainly fluctuation in the variants used as correspondences for the correct phonologic item in the target language where there are points of structural conflict between the native and target language, we can hardly conclude that they are unsystematic. Instead, we find a structured regularity that governs the fluctuation, and this regularity suggests a higher principle of language change. Language is a dynamic system, constantly undergoing change, and the way in which it changes follows a regular pattern, whether an entire system is changing its forms, a first language learner is acquiring the adult forms, or a second language learner is acquiring new forms. Ideally, the change moves from the categoric use of one form to another one, but the system passes through an orderly progression of variable stages as it goes from one extreme to the other. In second language learning, the stages are observed when a learner is required to learn a new unit in the second language. The orderly stages of progression in acquiring this unit can best be illustrated by taking the case of a typical "interference" variant and showing how it changes to the second language form. The model proposed here follows Wolfram (1978). For our illustrative purposes, we will take the case of the German speaker who is confronted with English [ə], in items such as *think, ether,* and *wreath.* German does not have the sound unit [ə], so the German speakers are confronted with acquiring this new phonologic form in the second language. Without a corresponding sound unit in German, speakers may use a unit from their native language in lieu of English [ə], and one of the common variants is [s], which is a unit in German.

In the first stage the use of [s] for [ə] may be categoric, so that [s] is always used in items such as *think* ([sɪŋk]), *ether* [isə] and *wreath* [ris]). In the next stage, we may begin to get [s] fluctuating with [ə] in a limited environment, perhaps only in word-initial position such as *think* [sɪŋk] and [əɪŋk]). Other environments, such as the intervocalic position of *ether* and the word-final position of *wreath,* would still evidence exclusive [s] use.

In the next stage, fluctuation between the correct English phone and the interference variant [s] may spread to a broader context, perhaps first to the intervocalic context of *ether* and then to the word-final position of *wreath.*

Following a stage of "maximal variability" (i.e., fluctuation in all environments), some environments will adopt the new variant categorically. Typically, this will taken place where the change to the new form was initiated originally. Thus, English [ə] may be adopted categorically in word-initial position, while continuing to fluctuate with [s] in intervocalic and final positions. Eventually, there is categorical adoption of the new variant in all the appropriate environments as the process of acquisition is completed. The logical stages of progression from the categorical use of the interference variant to the categorical acquisition of the new phone in the three environments is summarized in Table 3–1, where word-initial is E1, intervocalic E2, and word-final E3.

The model in this table provides an important starting point for seeing how new phonologic units in a second language are acquired. Naturally, this is an ideal; we know that many speakers' systems become "fossilized" so that they never complete the process of change. And, of course, the rate of passage from one stage to the next may vary greatly, so that no real-life time frame can be imposed on this progression. Nonetheless, we see that fluctuation occurs in a systematic way, constrained on the basis of different phonologic environments and moving in a regular progression from one stage to the next. Furthermore, different speakers go through the same stages in acquiring the new form.

An authentic model of second language phonologic acquisition will naturally have to represent additional dimensions of the interlanguage system. For instance, the notion of an "interference variant" needs some

Table 3–1. Stages in the Acquisition of a New Second Language Phonologic Unit

	E_1	E_2	E_3
Stage One (Categoric interference variant)	s	s	s
Stage Two (Limited variation)	s and ɵ	s	s
Stage Three (Expanded variation)	s and ɵ	s and ɵ	s
Stage Four (Maximal variation)	s and ɵ	s and ɵ	s and ɵ
Stage Five (Limited categorical adoption)	ɵ	s and ɵ	s and ɵ
Stage Six (Expanded categorical adoption)	ɵ	ɵ	s and ɵ
Stage Seven (Complete adoption)	ɵ	ɵ	ɵ

explanation. In the example in the table, it is suggested that the use of [s] for English [ɵ] was an interference form from the native language, based on our comparison of the two systems. Thus, equivalence between German [s] and English [ɵ] was assumed. But the notion of presumed equivalence between native and target language forms cannot always be predicted. In reality, some German speakers may use [t] instead of [s], or a given speaker may use both [t] and [s] for English [ɵ]. So, we cannot say that a single correspondence will always exist between the two language systems. For example, in one study of Japanese speakers producing the English consonant *r* (Dickerson and Dickerson, 1976), five different variants were observed, including the English target sound; and each of the ten subjects in the study showed the full range of variants indicated here:

Variants for English [r]
[ɾ] voiced nonretroflexed flap
[l] voiced lateral flap
[l] voiced lateral
[ɽ] voiced retroflexed flap
[r] voiced retroflexed semiconsonant

It is also necessary to clarify the nature of the relationship of phones in the native and target languages. We mentioned that the notion of equivalent structures in the native and target languages could not always be predicted, so that it is necessary to determine equivalence on an empirical basis. And, in the establishment of interference it is necessary to recognize productions that may be unique to the learner's system. In the study cited earlier, the range of phonetic variants reveals some productions that use phones in the native language, some that are phones in the target language, and some that may be unique to the learner's system. These unique sounds (which result as a product of interaction between systems) must be recognized as an authentic part of the interlanguage system.

In all of the preceding discussion, we have mentioned the important role of phonologic environment in determining variants. We may, for example, find a German speaker who uses [s] and [t] for English [θ] in initial position and [s] and [f] in final position. Or, the native Japanese speaker may use only [l] for English [r] preceding low vowels but [ɾ], [l], and [ɽ] before high vowels. The role of environment is important in determining the interlanguage variants that may occur and the range of fluctuation between variants. It should be noted that environment here must include all the dimensions found to be influential within any phonologic system, including the effect of neighboring sounds; the role of sounds in larger units such as syllables, words, and phrases; and prosodic features such as stress and intonation. Also, these different dimensions of environment may interact with each other, just as they may in a unitary phonologic system.

The model we propose here is one that accounts for the orderly progression from the units of one phonologic system to another. It takes into account the fluctuating nature of the interlanguage system while showing how the variability and change are highly systematic. Speakers of a new language do not suddenly awake with a new phonologic system. Instead, they go through an orderly progression of fluctuating variants, passing through inevitable stages as the process is carried to completion. In an important sense, the orderly acquisition of new forms in a second phonologic system recapitulates the process whereby all language systems undergo change.

PEDAGOGIC IMPLICATIONS

The treatment of second language learning problems within the context of speech and language pathology has engendered considerable controversy during the past several years. The basic issue concerns the responsibility of speech pathologists to treat such problems. Some (Bjarkman and Buckingham, 1981; Gandour 1980) have argued that second language learning problems are not appropriately treated in a clinical context because they do not involve disorders in the traditional application of this designation. Furthermore, these problems are not best handled by those techniques characteristic of a clinical setting. From this perspective, these problems should be left in the hands of those specifically educated in the methods of teaching English as a second language (TESL).

Others within speech pathology (Dreher, 1981; Gillcrist, 1981) have maintained that speech pathologists can assume responsibility for treating problems of the second language learner because of their education regarding communication problems of all types. Furthermore, there is no evidence that the traditional therapy methods employed by speech and language pathologists are inappropriate or inferior to those used by TESL specialists. In some instances, there is also a practical argument because the speech and language pathologist may be the only individual available for referral within a particular real-life setting.

Unfortunately, the dispute has sometimes been reduced to a question of professional territorial rights and the consequences of treating second language problems in training speech pathologists. (For example, there have been extended arguments over the validity of clinical "clock hours" obtained in assisting persons learning English as a second language). With due respect to the vested interests of different service professions and the genuine need to clarify certifiable clock hours in student clinical education, the issue seems to be somewhat misdirected. Instead of arguing over who has the right and obligation to handle such cases, we are better served by delimiting the requisite knowledge and pedagogic base for the individual engaged in such activities. The professional affiliation seems not nearly as important as the requisite qualifications.

Before the requisite knowledge base is set forth, it is necessary to reiterate our philosophic perspective on interlanguage. Repeatedly, we have referred to this kind of behavior as the norm for those learning a second language, so that a clinical designation as a "disorder" is inappropriate. Consideration of these problems as if they were no different from traditionally designated functional and organic disorders can only have negative attitudinal consequences. We must always bear in mind that we are dealing with a pedagogic problem, not a clinical one, and any practical approach to teaching phonology to learners to English as a second language must start from that vantage point.

Several dimensions of a requisite knowledge base derive from our earlier discussion of phonologic acquisition in a second language. First, it is necessary for the instructor to understand the comparative phonologies involved in the language learning situation. Such structural knowledge serves as the basis for understanding the kinds of phenomena that emerge in the interlanguage. Even those sounds that may be unique to the language learning situation are best viewed in terms of adaptive strategies that derive from the interaction of two language systems. It must be remembered here that the talker is not simply attempting to learn an English phonology, but attempting to learn this phonology on the basis of competence in another system with similarities to, and differences from, the target language. Understanding the points of structural similarity and difference thus becomes the starting point for focusing on the nature of the interlanguage system. The structural knowledge involved should include those aspects of the system discussed earlier, including the inventory of phonologic units, the phonotactic structures, and the various phonologic processes that operate in the respective phonologies. The instructor who starts with such contrastive knowledge is at considerable advantage in focusing on points of conflict that will lead to problems in the acquisition of the second language phonology. Practically speaking, this means that an instructor teaching English to a speaker of Spanish, Japanese, or German should know something about the structure of the respective phonologies, because the learner will encounter different problems in accordance with the native language system.*

A second requisite for the instructor involves analytic ability in describing a phonologic system. The system of the language learner must be analyzed on the basis of the observed interlanguage forms. This analytic ability starts with a practical knowledge of phonetics that allows the instructor to transcribe all the sounds produced by the learner in adequate detail, and extends to ability to describe the inventory of phonologic contrasts, phonotactics, and processes that are utilized by a given talker. All talkers are not at the same stage in their interlanguage, and accurate diagnosis is dependent upon the ability to understand each person's phonologic behavior as a system. The instructor needs to know the details of the phonologic system as a basis for setting up relevant instructional focus. Effective diagnosis, which is the reasonable basis for subsequent instruction, presumes this essential analytic ability.

---

*We distinguish here between structural knowledge of a language, which involves familiarity with its organizational patterns, and speaking knowledge, which involves proficiency in using the language as a means of communication.

A third base of knowledge involves understanding the nature of the second language learning process. In a sense, this understanding parallels the need to understand the native language acquisition process if a speech-language pathologist is to work with children acquiring the native language system. Important practical corollaries follow from understanding a model of second language acquisition. For example, given the important role of phonologic environment in influencing interlanguage variants and the progressive utilization of new forms in terms of these environments, phonologic context must figure prominently in the development of instructional materials. Similarly, fluctuation between variants is to be expected, and differing levels of fluctuation (in addition to different variants) should be expected in the acquisition process. If instructional materials are to recapitulate the normal progression of acquisition in a second language, then a viable model of this process must provide a base.

Finally, those dealing with second language learners should be familiar with the instructional strategies utilized in teaching the second phonology. In this respect, the field of TESL has developed particular strategies for developing students' perceptual and productive capabilities in another phonology. However, it should be noted that the basic methods in TESL and speech pathology are probably not as different as they sometimes appear on the surface. Thus, both speech pathologists and TESL teachers may set up discrimination tasks as a means of focusing on target phonologic units. Similarly, both may concern themselves with accurate phonetic production of target phones, utilizing various linguistic and nonlinguistic tasks to enhance the accurate production of the target phone. Also, both focus on aspects of linguistic and nonlinguistic "generalization" or "transfer," so that use in an increasingly broad range of phonologic contexts, and facility along an increasingly spontaneous continuum of extralinguistic situations, constitute an essential pedagogic concern. The details of tasks may be structured somewhat differently in speech pathology and TESL, but the underlying pedagogic principles are quite similar. Thus, the adaptation of the pedagogic approach should not be too imposing a task for a resourceful speech-language pathologist. In the final analysis, we must be more concerned with the requisite knowledge and pedagogic base of the individuals who teach a second phonology than with their professional affiliation. Second language learners stand to profit most from those who can apply appropriate descriptive, analytic, and pedagogic strategies regardless of their professional affiliation.

DIAGNOSIS AND REMEDIATION

For several reasons, issues of diagnosis and remediation are considerably more involved in an L2 than in an L1 system. Given the target norms of L2, it is essential to differentiate between a system differing from the target in accordance with the normal L2 phonologic acquisition process (i.e., *interlanguage norms*) and one which deviates from normal acquisition stages. The critical question is whether we can determine the difference between "normal" and "disordered" interlanguages, given that both will differ from the L2 target norms. The answer is complicated by several considerations related to the inherent nature of interlanguage. First, there is considerable fluctuation in how L2 target sounds may be modified. Thus, one speaker with a Vietnamese L1 background may use [t] for initial English [ɵ] and another may use [s], and both of these seem to be within normal limits. Furthermore, the same speaker may sometimes use [s] for [ɵ] and other times [t] for [ɵ] in the same item. This kind of fluctuation is a part of the normal developmental path, so that it is unrealistic to establish a unitary interlanguage norm.

Second, different persons may level or fossilize their interlanguage systems at varying stages. Thus, two persons with similar language backgrounds and similar exposure to the L2 may display quite different degrees of language transfer. While such differences indicate a range of proficiency levels in L2 acquisition, the situation seems relatively normal for interlanguage. Thus, we must recognize quite different individual proficiency levels within a broadly defined range of interlanguage normalcy.

Qualifications such as these certainly add complexity to an assessment task based on a developing L2 system. If the goal of the assessment is the identification of authentic phonologic disorders independent of language background, then assessment in the L1 certainly seems preferable. If this is not possible, then the assessment in L2 must proceed with the kinds of cautions discussed here. Realistic diversity in the interlanguage must be established as a baseline for assessment, just as normal dialectal variation must enter into the assessment of L1 clients with dialectally diverse backgrounds.

A speech-language pathologist called upon to serve a group for whom English is an L2 must usually accumulate data that can serve as a basis for establishing these kind of interlanguage norms. In many cases, the establishment of normal interlanguage for a particular group will have to be based on informal norms established by language-sensitive practitioners. For example, a speech pathologist asked to serve a Vietnamese refugee community will have to determine what the interlanguage norms are for that group. Thus, it may be determined that [t] and [s] for English initial [θ] are quite normal interlanguage norms based on an informal survey of talkers, but that an initial glottal stop [ʔ] for [θ] is not. From this perspective, the production of [sIn] or [tIn] for [θIn] would be considered normal, but [ʔIn] would not. Resourcefulness in such situations is obviously demanded, given the current scarcity of descriptions of L2 interlanguage systems, but the challenge seems appropriate for any speech pathologist serving such a population (Wolfram, 1979).

While the differentiation between normal interlanguage and disordered interlanguage looms important on a theoretical level, there is a practical point at which this issue may take a back seat to the practitioner's concern for basic intelligibility in the L2. When normal phonologic transfer imposes significant obstacles to intelligibility, then it seems appropriate for the speech pathologist to assist the development of the L2 phonology. The kinds of considerations that govern what aspects of the phonologic system are focused upon pedagogically, and the methods for modifying phonologic behavior, are not strikingly different in phonologic remediation and ESL training. For example, consider some of the factors that may enter into setting priorities for phonologic remediation:

1. The effect of pattern on intelligibility.
2. The generalization of the phonologic pattern.
3. The "functional load" of the phonologic opposition involved.
4. The fluctuation of the non-normative pattern.
5. The susceptibility to modification strategies.
6. The social obtrusiveness of the phonologic divergence.

These considerations may also serve the ESL teacher who adopts a systematic approach in setting priorities for developing phonologic materials in an L2.

The systematic organization of L2 pedagogy also parallels the classic considerations involved in the clinical approach to remediation in its concern for establishing the target behavior, generalizing the behavior linguistically and nonlinguistically, and stabilizing and retaining the behavior. A survey of remediation paradigms in speech pathology (e.g., Bernthal and Bankson, 1981; Winitz, 1975) and pedagogic approaches in ESL phonology (e.g., Goodman, 1980; Saville-Troike, 1976) finds many of the same kinds of drills, including techniques for phonetic establishment, discrimination, contrastive production, and generalization. If anything, the kinds of drills used in speech pathology are somewhat more exacting in pedagogic detail. Obviously, some adaptations will be made in ESL situations, given the dynamics of the systems involved. Thus, approaches to the treatment of underdifferentiation in L2 phonology may highlight discrimination training initially, whereas cases of phone substitution may focus on phonetic establishment. But even in these cases, similar strategies might derive from a comprehensive assessment of a phonologic disorder. In reality, then, the practical dimensions of L2 phonology seem quite susceptible to the traditional techniques utilized within the tradition of speech pathology. While the techniques designed to remediate phonologic disorders and to modify L2 interlanguage are common in many instances, there remains an important difference in perspective: divergence in L2 phonology is a normal part of the dynamics of adult second language learning, and any effort to increase proficiency in the L2 must highlight this normalcy rather than treat it as a basic disorder.

REFERENCES

Bernthal, J. E., and Bankson, N. W. (1981). *Articulation disorders.* Englewood Cliffs, NJ: Prentice-Hall.
Bjarkman, P. C., and Buckingham, H. W. (1981). A response to Gandour (Letter to the editor). *Journal of Speech and Hearing Disorders, 46,* 220.
Burt, M. K., and Kiparsky, C. (1972). The Gooficon: *A repair manual for English.* Rowley: Newbury House.
Corder, S. P. (1981). *Error analysis and interlanguage.* Oxford: Oxford University Press.
Dickerson, L. J., and Dickerson, W. B. (1976). Interlanguage phonology: Current trends and future directions. In S. P. Corder and E. Roulet (Eds.), *Actes du ème colloque de linguistique appliquèe de Neuchâtel.* Geneva: Universite de Neuchâtel.
Dreher, B. B. (1981). Response to Gandour (Letter to the editor). *Journal of Speech and Hearing Disorders, 46,* 217–218.
Dulay, H., and Burt, M. K. (1972). Goofing: An indication of children's second language learning strategies. *Language Learning, 22,* 235–252.
Gandour, J. (1980). Speech therapy and teaching English to speakers of other languages (Letter to the editor). *Journal of Speech and Hearing Disorders, 45,* 133–135.
Gillcrist, M. M. (1981). A rationale for providing service to the limited English proficiency student. *Language, Speech, and Hearing Services in Schools, 12,* 145–152.
Goodman, B. (1980). Improving foreigners' pronunciation of American English. ERIC No. ED 192 608.
Ingram, D. (1976). *Phonological disability in children.* London: Edward Arnold.
Macken, M. A., and Ferguson, C. A. (1981). Phonological universals in language acquisition. In H. Winitz (Ed.), *Native language and foreign language acquisition.* New York: New York Academy of Sciences.

Mulford, R., and Hecht, B. F. (1980). Learning to speak without an accent: Acquisition of a second language phonology. *Papers Representing Child Language Development, 18,* 16–74.

Oller, D. K. (1974). *Toward a general theory of phonological processes in first and second language learning.* Paper presented at the meeting of the Western Conference on Linguistics, Seattle.

Sato, C. J. (1983). *Phonological processes in second language acquisition: Another look at interlanguage syllable structure.* Paper presented at the 17th Annual TESOL Convention, Toronto.

Saville-Troike, M. (1976). *Foundations for teaching English as a second language: Theory and method for multicultural education.* Englewood Cliffs, NJ: Prentice-Hall.

Stampe, D. (1973). *A dissertation on natural phonology.* Unpublished doctoral dissertation, University of Chicago.

Tarone, E. (1976). Some influences on interlanguage phonology. *Working Papers in Bilingualism, 8,* 87–111.

Wardhaugh, R. (1970). The contrastive analysis hypothesis. *TESOL Quarterly, 4,* 124–129.

Weinreich, U. (1953). *Languages in contact.* The Hague, Netherlands: Mouton.

Winitz, H. (1975). *From syllable to conversation.* Baltimore: University Park Press.

Wode, H. (1977). The L2 acquisition of /r/. *Phonetica, 34,* 200–217.

Wolfram, W. (1978). Contrastive linguistics and social dialectology. *Language learning, 28,* 1–28.

Wolfram, W. (1979). *Dialect differences and speech pathology.* Washington, DC: Center for Applied Linguistics.

Wolfram, W. (1983). *Vietnamese English pronunciation.* Unpublished manuscript, Center for Applied Linguistics, Washington, DC.

Wolfram, W., and Johnson, R. (1982). *Phonological analysis: Focus on American English.* Washington, DC: Center for Applied Linguistics.

Part II
Voice

Chapter 4

Assessment and Treatment of Voice Disorders: State of the Art

William H. Perkins

In 1977, Paul Moore addressed the question of whether the major issues in voice disorders had been answered by research in speech science during the last 50 years. By way of softening his answer, which was "no," he reminded us that 300 years elapsed between the discovery of ether and its use as an anesthetic, 50 years between development of the laryngeal mirror and its use in diagnosis of laryngeal disease.

This is a review of what has been accomplished since 1976. (A "recent review" was operationally defined as work published during the last seven to eight years.) Although the answer for the voice clinician to Moore's question is still no, it is an answer that is changing rapidly in some areas. Of 170 articles reviewed, 132 were concerned with assessment and 38 with treatment, of which 27 described medical or surgical procedures for improving voice and only 11 dealt with voice therapy. As for assessment, of the 40 reports on acoustic methods, all but two involved detection of laryngeal pathology. Those two proposed an acoustic measure of vocal efficiency, the optimal target with which voice clinicians would presumably be primarily concerned, and both were written in German (Schultz-Coulon, Battmer, and Reichers, 1979).

By limiting this review to clinically relevant evidence (texts were included only if they reported data), what is presented is only the tip of the iceberg. With the growth of Japanese interest in voice science during the last decade, basic research in anatomy, physiology, and physics of voice has boomed, as has work in technology on measuring laryngeal function.

Two conferences on vocal fold physiology, one in 1980 at Kurume University, Japan, and the other in 1981 at the University of Wisconsin, provide a sense of the current frontiers. Topics ranged from the vascular network of the vocal fold, firing rate of motor units, neuromuscular control systems of phonation, and biorheology of vocal fold tissue to ultrasonic observation of vibratory action of inner layers of the vocal folds, computer simulations of cord vibration, interactions between glottal source and vocal tract, and relationships between glottal area time function and supraglottal pressure variation. Such topics as these, though not yet ready for clinical application, are all aspects of a common vocal mechanism that need basic understanding before a solid foundation for clinical application can be built (Stevens and Hirano, 1981). Unlike the 300 year delay for ether and the 50 years for the laryngeal mirror, clinical applications of voice research are already available for some aspects of assessment and are on the horizon for other problems of voice.

ASSESSMENT

Technology of Measurement

The development of instruments for measuring vocal function has attracted the largest body of scientific advances that are clinically useful. A conference organized by the Communicative Disorders Program of the National Institute of Neurological and Communicative Disorders and Stroke (NINCDS) in 1979 points up the priority of this area of advancement. The purpose of the conference was to identify objective, reliable, valid procedures for assessing voice disorders, which can permit communication of findings among clinics and clinical investigators. The voice scientists, speech pathologists, and laryngologists who participated concluded that fiberoptic, electromyographic, airflow, acoustic, and laryngographic techniques were highly relevant to the assessment of neurologic dysfunction, vocal cord lesions, morphologic changes of the cords, and abnormal phonatory function. They also concluded, however, that no technique could be singled out as the most effective (Ludlow and Hart, 1982).

Assessment of Laryngeal Pathology

Table 4–1 summarizes the assessment needs addressed by this conference. Judging from frequency of use in studies reported, acoustic

Table 4-1. Types of Measures Needed in the Management of Vocal Pathologies

Clinical Service	Measures Needed
Detection of changes in laryngeal tissues following completion of radiation treatment for laryngeal carcinoma.	Measures of changes in the stiffness and mass of the cords as may be reflected in phonatory functioning.
Assessment and reassessment of vocal nodules during voice therapy.	Objective, standardized, and reliable measures of the size and position of nodules from visual recordings. Measures of the effects of vocal nodules on phonatory function. Measures of differences in vocal cord positioning and vibratory patterns which may contribute to the development of the nodules.
Assessment and reassessment of recurrent laryngeal paresis/paralysis; abductor paresis/paralysis; superior laryngeal paresis/paralysis.	Objective, standardized, and reliable graphic measures of resting, inspiratory, and adducted positioning of the cords. Measures of vocal efficiency and range of phonatory functioning. Measures of muscle fiber activity in the vocalis, interarytenoid, posterior cricoarytenoid, and cricothyroid.
Diagnosis and assessment of "functional" phonatory disorders.	Measures of degree and type of deviation from normal in: Vocal cord positioning. Vibratory patterns. Patterns of intrinsic and extrinsic muscle fiber firing at rest and during phonation. Relative timing of adductor-abductor antagonistic muscle group contractions.
Assessment and reassessment of phonatory disorders associated with neuromuscular disorders.	Measures of degree and type of deviation from normal in: Muscle fiber firing at rest and during contraction. Synchronization of onset of firing in adductor and abductor muscle antagonists. Vibratory cycle. The rate of positioning of the vocal cords for phonation onset and offset during connected speech.
Detection of changes in esophageal speech which may be signs of carcinoma reoccurrence.	Measures of changes in: Rate of syllable production. Airflow during speech. Vocal efficiency for intensity. Median and range in fundamental frequency. Extraneous noise production during speech.

Ludlow, C. L. (1982). Research needs for the assessment of phonatory function. In C. L. Ludlow and M. O. Hart (Eds.), *Proceedings of the Conference on the Assessment of Vocal Pathology* (ASHA Reports 11) (p. 5). Rockville, MD: American Speech-Language-Hearing Association.

measures are the preferred technique for meeting as many of these needs as possible. This is not surprising, considering that these measures are nonintrusive, can be gathered and analyzed relatively easily, permit calibration and quantification, and provide inferences for a wide range of interpretations of normal and abnormal laryngeal conditions and patterns of vibration.

Acoustic Measures. Acoustic studies reported since 1976 have been concerned with two clinical topics: detection of pathologic laryngeal conditions and assessment of voice quality. In an excellent review, Davis (1979, 1982) analyzed various acoustic measures available and the clinical uses to which they can be put.

The underlying premise for detection of laryngeal pathology is that a deviant condition will result in an acoustic "signature" affecting fundamental frequency, intensity, or quality, singly or in combination. Pathology that affects vocal fold mass, elasticity, stiffness, or length will affect fundamental frequency. Paralysis of respiratory or laryngeal musculature will reduce sufficiency of subglottal pressure and, accordingly, of vocal intensity. The traditional early warning sign of laryngeal pathology, hoarseness, is heard as a deviant quality but can also involve fundamental frequency and intensity. A tumor or parlysis of one cord that produces asymmetric mass, stiffness, or elasticity will cause asymmetric cord vibration with consequent breathiness, reduced intensity, pitch perturbation (jitter), and amplitude perturbation (shimmer).

Much of the recent effort to detect pathology acoustically has used indirect rather than direct signals. The problem with direct signals is the resonance effect of the vocal tract, which, along with the glottal source component, constitutes the radiated sound. It is the glottal component, of course, which is affected by laryngeal pathology. Throat contact microphones, one type of direct signal that minimizes vocal tract resonances, also present problems: intervening neck tissue functions as a low pass filter, and the signal is sensitive to microphone placement. These difficulties have led to the use of a long metal reflectionless tube to separate the glottal source from resonance effects of the vocal tract. Although simple and inexpensive, it requires vocal tract adjustments that raise questions about the validity of the procedure (Monsen, 1982).

The more frequently used approach is *inverse filtering,* which requires computer analysis to filter out supraglottal resonance contributions to the signal. What remains is a more useful approximation of the glottal signal, which can be analyzed for effects of laryngeal pathology. Two methods of inverse filtering have been used. *Glottal inverse filtering* now uses digital computer techniques to estimate formant frequencies and band widths from which all but the glottal wave form is supposed to be removed. The resulting wave form, however, does not correspond satisfactorily with concepts of vocal cord closure (Davis, 1982; Hiki, Imazzumi, Hirano, Matsushita, and Kakita, 1976).

The other indirect method is *residue inverse filtering.* It is the inverse of the estimated lip radiation, vocal tract, and glottal spectral contributions to the speech signal. The signal that remains exhibits strong peaks at the start of each pitch period. The *residue* signal is obtained with a phase-insensitive autocorrelational method, which does not require the visual inspection of formants, marking of pitch periods, or controlled recording conditions necessary for glottal inverse filtering. Thus, the residual signal, although more of an abstraction than the glottal signal, is easier to obtain and has greater potential value for detecting laryngeal pathology (Davis, 1982; Markel and Gray, 1976). Although in some intermediate or advanced cases it does not seem to provide more information about the pathology than the unfiltered speech signal, in other early cases it has detected pathology that was not otherwise apparent (Davis, 1976).

Earlier work on acoustic effects of laryngeal pathology on periodicity of vocal cord vibration has continued (Kitajima and Gould, 1976; Murry and Doherty, 1980). Several approaches have been used. *Pitch period perturbation* is the time difference between durations of successive pitch periods in the vocal tone. Relative average perturbation, taking into account the slow smooth changes in pitch period that occur normally, provides a smoothed trend line against which rapid erratic perturbations can be measured. This measure has been refined into a frequency perturbation quotient (FPQ). Fundamental frequency perturbation, taking account of greater normal perturbation at higher frequencies, has provided a basis for distinguishing effects of laryngeal cancer between male and female voices. *Amplitude perturbation* is determined by correlograms of a series of amplitude values at each pitch period peak. This measure has been developed as an amplitude perturbation quotient (APQ). More recently, Davis (1976, 1982) used the residue signal, rather than the unfiltered speech signal, to devise an automated procedure for determining pitch and amplitude perturbation quotients (PPQ and APQ), which improve discrimination of pathologic from normal voice. Recognizing that the signal-to-noise ratio is higher between pitch peaks of the residue signal of pathologic than of normal voices, and that detection of fundamental frequency is made difficult by the "breathy" voice caused by pathology, Davis (1976) has also developed acoustic measures using these characteristics.

How to interpret pitch perturbation as evidence of pathology is confounded by its occurrence in normal voices (Horii, 1979). Exactly why it is greater in pathologic larynges is not entirely clear (Koike, Takahashi, and Calcaterra, 1977). For that matter, although earlier studies reported a relationship between perception of pathology and pitch perturbation, more recent work shows a negative relationship (Horii, 1979; Ludlow, 1982; Nichols, 1979).

Spectral analysis is another acoustic basis for detection of laryngeal pathology (Kitajima, 1981). Investigations over the last two decades have shown noise components in pathologic voices that mask formant and fundamental frequency characteristics. Observing that spectral flatness increases with spectral noise, Davis (1976) developed spectral measures for vocal assessment. Using features and signals obtained with residue inverse filtering, he developed a voice profile with which normal and pathologic voices can be differentiated. Although spectral flatness measures were useful in making the distinction, perturbation quotients were better, but still not infallible.

Spectrographic analysis has been used to study the breathiness of abductor spastic dysphonia and the strained voice arrests of adductor spastic dysphonia (Merson and Ginsberg, 1979; Wolfe and Bacon, 1976). Similarly, some correlations have been found between spectral characteristics and such voice qualities as overtight-breathy, hyper-hypokinetic, and nasality (Fritzell, Hammarberg, and Wedin, 1977; Gauffin and Sundberg, 1977; Lindblom, Lubker, and Pauli, 1977; Wirz, Subtelny and Whitehead, 1981).

Attractive as the potential of acoustic measures is for detecting laryngeal pathology, Ludlow (1982) points out that with the current state of knowledge, acoustic screening methods are not yet feasible. What these measures detect is hoarseness and roughness, qualities frequently found in voices not necessarily affected by pathology (Brindle and Morris, 1979; Emanuel and Austin, 1981; Emanuel and Scarzini, 1979, 1980; Hanson and Emanuel, 1979; Whitehead and Lieberth, 1979). Thus, until functional hoarseness can be reliably differentiated from pathologic hoarseness, acoustic methods will not become realistic tools of clinical assessment. Still, Hirano, Hiki, Imazzumi, Kakita, and Matsushita (1978) have demonstrated in a preliminary study of 217 patients with various pathologies that 84 per cent of them could be separated from 20 normal subjects. Similarly, 84 per cent of the cancer patients could be differentiated from those with other pathologies, and 70 per cent of patients with polyps, sulcis vocalis, and recurrent laryngeal paralysis could be differentiated. In a similar study of 30 patients, using long-term speech spectra, comparable results were obtained (Wendler, Doherty, Hollien, 1980). Whether their multivariate analysis of spectral harmonics, frequency perturbation, and amplitude perturbation will meet Ludlow's reservations remains to be determined.

Nonacoustic Measures. Various other measures have received recent attention as being clinically useful. What is searched for are quantitative measures of degree of laryngeal impairment that can provide a basis for comparison with the normal (Ludlow, 1982). Some have been in use for years; others seem to hold great potential but have barely been explored in laryngeal studies.

Ultrasound, the use of which has burgeoned in many areas of medicine, seems to have advantages for laryngeal inquiry. Using the principle of sonar, high frequency sound is reflected from internal structures that differ in acoustic reflective properties such as soft and hard tissues, fluids, and gases. Presumably, ultrasound could provide a nonintrusive method of visualizing the larynx, but extensive research will be needed before clinical merits can emerge (Hamlet, 1982).

Video nasopharyngoscopy has been used to visualize cord action in dysarthric speech (Ludlow and Bassich, 1981). A similar device, the laryngeal fiberscope with the lens positioned just below the velum, is routinely used in Japan for laryngeal diagnosis (Andrews, 1977; Fujimura, 1982; Parnes, Lavarato, and Myers, 1978; Sawashima, 1976). It has also been used with stroboscopic light (Gould, Kojima, and Labiase, 1979; Saito, Fukuda, Kitahara, and Kokawa, 1978). The most recent advance is a stereofiberscope that permits three-dimensional visualization of the larynx (Fujimura, Baer, and Niimi, 1979). An alternative method of visualizing laryngeal pathology is computerized tomography. With reduced cost and radiation, the better information it provides makes it competitive with cinelaryngoscopy and laryngography (Ward, Hanafee, Mancuso, and Shallit, 1979). One of the costs in high speed cinematography, frame-by-frame analysis time, has been reduced with a video scanning technique for extracting glottal measurements (Childers, Paige, and Moore, 1976). On a much simpler and more practical level, a concave laryngeal mirror has been developed that magnifies and brightens the image (Janfaza, 1978).

Because air wastage tends to characterize laryngeal pathology and motor speech disorders, measures of *laryngeal management of the breath stream* are of clinical interest (Kelman, Gordon, Morton, and Simpson, 1981). Several noninvasive methods have been used. *Airflow wave form* at the vocal folds can be obtained from the oral air flow at the mouth with an inverse filter technique as well as with a refinement of the traditional pneumotachographic technique. A relatively simple clinical procedure for measuring *laryngeal airway resistance* has been developed (Merson and Ginsberg, 1979; Rothenberg, 1977, 1982; Smitheran and Hixon, 1981). Similarly, Forner and Hixon (1977) have simplified a kinematic method of measuring speech breathing that requires little training of clinician or client; is safe, precise, and rapid; and permits natural speech in real time. From an oscilloscopic display, changes of chest wall, and rib cage and abdomen contributions to lung volume, can be examined.

Whereas glottal air flow mainly reflects vocal fold movements when the glottis is open, *vocal fold contact area* yields information about the period of glottal closure. This information has been obtained with a laryngograph, a term preferred to glottograph. What is measured is current between electrodes on each side of the larynx. Current flow varies directly with the area of contact between the cords (Askenfelt, Gauffin, Sundberg, and Kitzing, 1980; Rothenberg, 1982; Teany, 1980).

Fourcin (1982) has presented evidence showing how laryngograph output can be analyzed to discriminate among pathologies and between normal and pathologic function. On the premise that different pathologies involve different vocal fold contacts, what the laryngograph presumably yields is a record of the performance of the vocal folds as they prepare to release acoustic pulses. Whether this record can overcome the difficulties of acoustic analysis and provide a basis for discriminating functional aperiodic vibration from pathologic aperiodicity remains to be determined. A difficulty that has often been encountered is the weakness of the signal obtained from some talkers (Rothenberg, 1982). Equally troubling in a comparison of laryngographic and stroboscopic measures of glottal openings and closings were wide variability and low correlations between the measures (Pederson, 1977).

Electromyography is another traditional tool that has been used in many studies of normal laryngeal function, but unlike its use with neuromuscular disorders, it has not been used for diagnosis of laryngeal muscle performance (Guidi, Bannister, Gibson, and Payne, 1981; Harris, 1982). Beyond its relevance for determining abnormalities of laryngeal motor firing, it may also prove essential to the determination of patterns of muscular contraction of functional dysphonia as they are distinguished from patterns of optimal vocal production.

Behavioral Measurement

For clinicians who have limited equipment, reliable behavioral procedures for assessing laryngeal functioning would be particularly useful. Only two studies of adults that address this need have been reported in the last five years. Gordon, Morton, and Simpson (1978) found that patients with additive laryngeal lesions had considerably reduced phonation times for some sustained vowels. These glottal margin tumors, such as nodules and polyps, presumably interfere with efficient cord closure. The consequences are decreased laryngeal airway resistance, increased air flow, and reduced phonation time.

As an indicator of adequacy of laryngeal function, an s/z ratio was devised and tested on 28 subjects with nodules or polyps, 36 dysphonic subjects with no laryngeal pathology, and 86 normally speaking subjects (Eckel and Boone, 1981). No differences were found among these groups in ability to sustain /s/. Similarly, normal speakers did not sustain /z/ much longer than did dysphonic speakers with no pathology, nor did their s/z ratios differ much from 1.0. The pathologic speakers differed significantly from both of these groups by ratios in excess of 1.4 95 per cent of the time, and by shorter durations of /z/. It should be noted, however, that some subjects from both nonpathologic groups showed shorter durations of /z/ and larger s/z ratios than did most of the pathologic subjects. Still, this behavioral screening measure is the most useful yet developed.

Voice Disorder Characteristics

With any disorder, assessment and treatment are dependent on the understanding of it. Most of the recent work on voice disorders has been concerned with the nature of the problems. Although it has not yet culminated in valid and reliable clinical methods, it is the forerunner of the development of such methods. Because it may soon result in the development of assessment procedures, it is reviewed in this section.

Spastic Dysphonia

In 1976, Dedo reported sectioning the recurrent laryngeal nerve as a treatment of spastic dysphonia. Whatever the ultimate merits of this procedure, its indisputable effect was that more recent inquiry has been devoted to this voice disorder than to any other. Whereas traditionally it was mainly considered to be a psychogenic disorder (Brodnitz, 1976), the tide of research abruptly swung to viewing it as a neuropathology. Because control of laryngeal muscle is related to that of middle ear muscles, acoustic reflexes as well as laryngeal nerves and muscles have been investigated (McCall, 1977). Although evidence of histopathology in the recurrent laryngeal nerve has been reported, other evidence has been negative (Aminoff, Dedo, and Izdebski, 1978; Bocchino and Tucker, 1978; Dedo, Izdebski, and Townsend, 1977; Dedo, Townsend, and Izdebski, 1978; Izdebski, 1977; Ravits, Aronson, DeSanto, and Dyck, 1979). Similarly, acoustic reflex differences have been found by some but not by others (Hall and Jerger, 1976; Sharbrough, Stockard, and Aronson, 1978). Still others have suspected focal dystonia of laryngeal musculature (Aminoff et al., 1978).

The meaning of this flurry of interest was the subject of a state-of-the-art conference in 1979 (Lawrence, 1979). The idea that spastic dysphonia is basically a neuropathology is attractive, but no one is certain whether the pathology, if it exists, is peripheral or central. Definitive answers are not yet available. A difficulty with accounting for a spastic condition with peripheral nerve pathology is that the symptom should be flaccidity rather than spasticity.

Perhaps the explanation, at least in part, lies in the evidence of two types of intermittent dysphonia, which in one case were both found in the same patient (Cannito and Johnson, 1981). Traditionally, spastic dysphonia is characterized by adductor spasms, resulting in intermittent strangulation of phonation that resembles essential voice tremor (Aronson and Hartman, 1981). By contrast, several patients have been reported with intermittent abductory spasms. Because the laryngeal behavior is different and the causes may be different, some have resisted the classification "spastic dysphonia—abductor type." Preferred alternatives are "intermittent abductory dysphonia" or "intermittent breathy dysphonia" (Bacon and Wolfe, 1980; Hartman and Aronson, 1981; Merson and Ginsberg, 1979; Parnes et al., 1978; Shipp, Mueller, and Zwitman, 1980; Zwitman, 1979). Whether the neuropathology of one is peripheral, and of the other is central, has not been established.

Motor Voice Disorders

Dysphonic effects of the various dysarthrias are often a consequence of difficulty in initiating and terminating phonation for onset and offset of voice during connected speech, especially in Parkinson's disease. Also affected in Shy-Drager syndrome, myasthenia gravis, Wilson's disease, amyotrophic lateral sclerosis, and tardive dyskinesia, as well as in Parkinson's disease, are abilities to control pitch, loudness, and quality (Dordain and Chevrie-Muller, 1977; Logemann, Fisher, Boshes, and Blonsky, 1978; Ludlow, 1982; Ludlow and Bassich, 1981; Portnoy, 1979; Williams, Hanson, and Calne, 1979). The involuntary grunting and throat-clearings of Gilles de la Tourette syndrome are among the less obtrusive symptoms of this bizarre disorder, which include coprolalia, echolalia, multiple tics, and involuntary jumping, squatting, and kicking. The cause of this dramatic disorder is uncertain, although recent evidence suggests a neurologic basis, a possibility supported by the tendency of affected children to have learning disabilities (Cohen, Shaywitz, Caparulo, Young, and Bowers, 1978; Golden, 1977).

Laryngeal Pathology

Some work has been done relating laryngeal function to voice disorders (Moore, 1976). Murry (1978) has shown that with the exception of a narrowed pitch range in laryngeal paralysis, fundamental frequency is not systematically different in laryngeal pathology from normal, perceptual impressions notwithstanding.

Paralysis. Frequently, a paralyzed vocal fold lies higher than the healthy one. Experimentation with simulated contraction of the lateral cricoarytenoid muscle suggests that this arytenoid displacement can be corrected (Baken and Isshiki, 1977). In somewhat surprising results of experimentation on the excised larynx, the effect of asymmetric tension in the vocal cords turned out opposite to expectation (Isshiki, Tanabe, Ishizaka, and Broad, 1977). Presumably, as cord tension increases, amplitude of vibration decreases. In computer simulation of this physiologic experiment, however, it was found that the tense cord (simulating the healthy cord) vibrated with somewhat greater amplitude than the "paralyzed" lax cord. Moreover, the lax cord dominated the tense one in determining pitch. Despite asymmetric tension (a simulation of unilateral paralysis), if the two cords started from a closed position, they vibrated at the same frequency, even though the tense cord opened faster and then had to wait for the lax cord to catch up. Thus, asymmetric tension alone did not result in hoarseness (Ishizaka and Isshiki, 1976; Isshiki, 1977a).

The implication of these experiments for clinical management of laryngeal paralysis is that if impaired cord resistance is not overpowered with excessive breath pressure, thereby permitting cord closure between vibratory cycles, a reasonably clear voice can be obtained. This brings into question the appropriateness of the widespread "effort" techniques intended to obtain reflexive closure of the cords by effortful lifting, pushing, coughing, or grunting. All of these procedures generate high levels of subglottal pressure, which would work against complete cord closure between cycles. Conversely, the clinical approach supported by this research is to strive for clear tone at a level of loudness as reduced as is necessary to obtain it. With clear tone, the clinician has evidence of symmetric cord vibration with each cycle, presumably beginning from a condition of closure.

Functional Pathology. Pivotal research has been concerned with the nature of vocal cord stress and its significance for vocal abuse in the development of functional pathology. In meticulous preliminary research, Hirano, Kurita, Matsuo, and Nagata (1980, 1981) have studied vocal fold reactions to stress that lead to acute inflammation, subepithelial bleeding, nodules, contact granulomas, polyps, and polypoid degeneration (Reinike's edema). They confirmed that all of these pathologies are largely a consequence of vocal abuse, with the exception of polypoid vocal fold.

Although polypoid hypertrophy is often thought to be basically similar to the polyp, it is not. Characterized by a chronic edematous lesion extending the length of the membranous vocal fold, usually bilaterally, polypoid hypertrophy appears to be caused primarily by smoking and age. Vocal abuse can aggravate the condition, but it is not likely to cause it. These conclusions are based on observations of 57 male and 40 female subjects. In 88 per cent, hoarseness did not begin until age 40, and then it progressed so slowly that most patients did not seek medical help for one to three years. Over three fourths of the patients smoked at least half a pack of cigarettes a day; otherwise, less than half showed any predisposing conditions such as excessive vocal abuse, air pollution, drinking, or the common cold.

Polyps and polypoid swelling both form in the superficial layer of the lamina propria. (The lamina propria of the mucosa, just beneath the thin epithelial surface of the cord, has three layers. The superficial layer is loose and pliable, with few fibers; the intermediate layer is composed chiefly of elastic fibers; and the deep layer consists mainly of collagenous thread-like fibers. The two deeper layers constitute the vocal ligament.) They differ, however, in form, location, and cause. Polyps develop as pedunculated tumors, ranging in size from small to large, attached to the middle of the membranous cord. Judging from data on 629 patients, polyps occur mainly in middle age, rarely in childhood, and somewhat more frequently in male than in female patients. They appear to be caused by a traumatic lesion of small vessels in the lamina propria during abusive phonation, often following a common cold. Neither smoking nor drinking appears to be much involved in causation. Apparently, mechanical stresses of deep layers of cord vibration rupture venules, which hemorrhage, giving the inital reddish appearance that changes to white as the hemorrhages in the polyp become old.

Nodules also develop in the superficial layer of the lamina propria, and at the same location on the cord as polyps. Mechanical vibratory stress in the nodule, however, appears confined to the cord edge, which is free of blood vessels, and activates proliferation of fibroblasts that produce collagenous fibers, which thicken the epithelium to form the whitish mass of the nodule. In 309 cases of nodule, no significant pathology of blood vessels was observed.

The relationship of age and sex to nodular development is somewhat puzzling. In children, far more boys than girls develop nodules, presumably because they yell more. In adults, nodules are rarely found in males, at least in Japan, but are as prevalent in middle aged women as in young boys. Polyps, on the other hand, are more frequently found in low pitch males than in high pitch females. This has led to the speculation that high pitches activate cord edge stress, leading to nodules, whereas low pitches activate deep layer stress, which ruptures blood vessels and causes polyps. How this explanation would account for polyps when they do occur in high-pitched women or nodules in adult low-pitch males has not been determined.

Hirano and colleagues (1980) differentiated acute from chronic reactions to vocal abuse, with nodules, polyps, and contact ulcers being chronic manifestations. Acute inflammation is a typical reaction to temporary excessive vocal abuse, such as yelling at a football game. The superficial layer of the lamina propria becomes edematous from leakage of serum and dilation of blood vessels. With increased stress, blood vessels rupture, resulting in subepithelial bleeding. Both of these acute conditions subside within a week or two of vocal rest and easy quiet phonation. Inflammation, the most frequent problem of professional speakers and singers, can also result from hormonal imbalance, such as that occurring during menstruation in some women, and upper respiratory infection (Schiff and Gould, 1978).

The effects of androgen on mutational voice change were studied in 35 cases of eunuchoidism. Treatment to lower the pitch to normal took 6 months to 2 years. Surprisingly, pitch changes often preceded structural development of the larynx. Apparently, mutational voice change may occur as a result of mode of laryngeal adjustments and changes in soft tissue (Hirose, Sawashima, Ushijima, and Kumamoto, 1977).

Respiration

Hixon, Mead, and Goldman (1976) and Forner and Hixon (1977) have pioneered in definitive studies of speech respiration. Among their recent contributions are investigations of the thorax, rib cage, diaphragm, and abdomen in normal and hearing impaired speech. In normal conversational speech, abdominal forces tune the diaphragm to facilitate minimal interruption of ongoing speech for needed inspiratory pauses. Respiration function in the hearing impaired differed from normal in several ways, including deviance in lung volume adjustments as well as in laryngeal and upper airway adjustments.

Comparisons have also been made of respiration in trained and untrained subjects (Baken, 1979; Baken and Cavallo, 1979, 1981; Proctor, 1979; Wilder, 1979). Although the rib cage and the diaphragm-abdomen, which are the two components of the chest wall, are linked within limits, they also can function independently. Thus, knowledge of the volume of air expired does not reveal relative activity of rib cage or abdomen. Presumably, an unlimited number of rib cage–abdominal patterns could be used to achieve the lung volumes and pressures needed for phonation. To the contrary, well defined prephonatory chest-wall adjustments were found in both trained and untrained talkers. They seem to represent an innate adjustment that has evolved to facilitate phonation. Trained subjects did differ in several ways, however, one of which was wider variations in patterns of chest wall adjustment.

Phonatory Control

Control of any phonatory episode involves the following sequence: prephonatory inspiration, which provides the necessary lung volume for the phrase of an intended length, loudness, pitch, and quality; prephonatory expiration and prephonatory tuning of the vocal folds for the intended utterance; phonatory expiration and modulation of laryngeal activity; and monitoring of the vocal output. Modulation of laryngeal activity is accomplished with three intrinsic reflexogenic systems, with receptors in the mucosa, joints, and muscles. The mucosal and muscle receptors are sensitive to the stretching force of expiratory pressure, whereas mechanoreceptors in the joints mediate cartilage adjustments during phonation (Gould, 1979; Wyke, 1979).

The role of feedback in voice control has also been studied in relation to nasality and laryngeal sensation (Garber and Moller, 1979; Horii and Weinberg, 1979; Leonard and Ringel, 1979; Sorenson, Horii, and Leonard, 1980; Stevens, Nickersen, Boothroyd, and Rollins, 1976). With normally hearing subjects, nasality has been shown to be under auditory feedback control. Lacking auditory feedback, visual feedback has been used to reduce nasality in the deaf. Presumably, phonatory control should be impaired by anesthetization of laryngeal mucosa. Although jitter increases as a result, especially at high frequencies, ability to match pitches was not affected in earlier experiments. Approaching the phonatory control system from a test of auditory and somesthetic feedback times, both sensory modalities were stimulated to determine minimal reaction times for phonatory initiation (Izdebski and Shipp, 1978). This novel tracking task placed greater dynamic demands on the mucosal feedback system, which, when anesthetized, resulted in impaired performance.

Talker Characteristics of Voice

A variety of vocal characteristics of talkers have been investigated, ranging from sex differences and effects on voice of smoking to perceptual systems of voice description. The area of greatest interest, however, has been the effects of age on voice.

Aging

Aside from voice disorders that are characteristic of various ages, such as mutational problems of adolescence and polyps of middle age, aging has effects on the voice that can be detected by observers. A fundamental difficulty in studying vocal aging is in how to define it. Should it be in terms of chronological age or in terms of decrement of vocal function? What should be the measures of perceptual, acoustic, physiologic, and anatomic characteristics? If aging effects are as variable as suspected, which populations should be studied? With these issues still unresolved, work in this area has been mostly exploratory and descriptive (Brodnitz, 1978; Weinberg, 1978; Wilder, 1978).

Beginning with preadolescence, the current description of voice at various ages is as follows. Because girls mature faster than boys, they approach adolescence with slightly lower speech-fundamental frequencies, (SFF), although a recent study suggests the opposite (Hasek, Singh, and Murry, 1980). During adolescence, their SFF becomes gradually lower until adulthood, at which time it remains essentially level until after menopause, when it lowers. In male subjects, who have been studied far more than female subjects, SFF drops about an octave in four to five years during puberty, then continues to lower gradually until about age 40, at which time it begins to rise slowly through the declining years. Pitch range increases during puberty, at least in males, and then declines in the aged. Some elderly voices exhibit tremor, breathiness, pitch variability, increased loudness, and increased noise at the expense of clear tone. Doubt has been cast, however, on jitter and shimmer as the reasons why aged voices are perceived as noisy and rough. Surprisingly, speed of speech is not reduced with age, but precision in achieving speech targets at fast rates is diminished (Hanley, Hanson, and Miller, 1978; Hartman, 1979; Hollien, 1978; Hollien and Tolhurst, 1978; Horii and Ryan, 1981; Horii and Weinberg, 1979; Stoicheff, 1981; Sweeting, 1979; Weinberg, 1978; Wilder, 1978).

This pattern must be recognized as being preliminary. Wide individual variations from it seem abundant, but little is known of these variations. For that matter, because of relatively few investigations, little is known of the female voice. What is known points to greater changes with age in the male than the female.

Recent histologic and laryngoscopic studies may account for some of these changes. Ossification and calcification of the larynx have been found to begin earlier and to be more extensive in male subjects than female subjects. In senility, men's vocal folds tend to atrophy, whereas those of women show mainly edema. That could explain why pitch becomes higher in the former and lower in the latter (Honjo and Isshiki, 1980; Kahane, 1980).

Perceptual Systems of Voice

Three approaches to the perceptual analysis of voice have been taken recently. Colton and Estill (1976, 1978) and Colton, Estill, and Gould (1977), in devising a system for categorizing voice quality, selected four qualities that could be perceptually distinguished: speech (as in everyday conversation), cry, twang, operatic ring. Their objective was to determine the acoustic and physiologic characteristics of these perceptual modes in order to fully describe the various qualities of the human voice.

In multidimensional analyses designed to differentiate between abnormal and normal voices, listeners used more dimensions to judge differences among pathologic voices than normal ones. Apparently, the perceptual strategy for judging normal voices of both sexes is to sort them according to sex and then make separate judgements for male and female subjects, possibly according to cultural stereotypes. Male subjects were judged for similarity on the basis of effort, pitch, and hoarseness; female subjects were characterized by effort, pitch, and nasality (Murry and Singh, 1980; Murry, Singh, and Sargent, 1977; Singh and Murry, 1978).

The third approach represents an attempt to delineate in measurable dimensions all of the independent perceptual elements by which vocal production is controlled. The purpose of this effort is to obtain the acoustic correlates of these perceptual dimensions that, by themselves, are impossible to verify and are very difficult, if not impossible, to measure reliably in a wide range of subjects (Ludlow, 1982). With acoustic correlates of these dimensions established, vocal production can be experimentally manipulated to determine patterns of vocal abuse and vocal efficiency (Perkins, 1978).

Sex Characteristics

Fundamental frequency, sound pressure level, and quality have been studied in male, female, and male transsexual subjects. The slight hoarseness that is reported in trained female singers during menstruation, presumably because of vocal fold edema, was not found in voices of normal untrained female subjects, possibly because they did not perform comparably strenuous vocal tasks (Schiff, 1977; Silverman and Zimmer, 1978). In another investigation, fundamental frequency-sound pressure level (f_O-SPL) profiles of young adult male and female subjects with normal voices were compared for maximum and minimum SPL with 10 per cent intervals of f_O. Male and female subjects were similar in f_O range, SPL output throughout f_O range, and SPL range. The profile has potential for graphing the range of frequencies at which the voice functions most efficiently.

In other experiments, fundamental frequency and vocal tract resonance were studied for their contribution to the perception of femaleness in the voice. In natural speech, f_O was the major determinant in one study, but in another, vocal tract resonance played a major role. On the other hand, in the case of a male transsexual subject who had undergone hormone therapy and had raised her pitch, her voice was still discernibly different from a natural female voice. Interestingly, when trying to sound sexy, both males and females use lower pitches as well as slower rates (Bralley, Bull, and Gore, 1978; Brown and Feinstein, 1977; Coleman, 1976; Coleman, Mabis, and Hinson, 1977; Tuomi and Fisher, 1979).

Other Talker Characteristics

Isolated investigations of talker characteristics have ranged from vocal cues of schizophrenia to effects of a dental prosthesis on voice. In the latter study, use of an experimental dental appliance altered personal characteristics of voice to varying degrees for both listeners and speakers. In the former, schizophrenic talkers were differentiated from nonschizophrenic talkers, probably on the basis of vocal qualities, particularly flat inflection. Voice characteristics of depressive patients did not change significantly with treatment (Darby and Hollien, 1977; Hamlet, Geoffrey, and Bartlett, 1976; Todt and Howell, 1980; Tuomi and Fisher, 1979).

Two other studies were concerned with pitch and loudness. One tested the observation that talkers sound different to themselves than to listeners. Although this may be true for some aspects of voice, it is apparently not true in the perception of pitch. In the other, an investigation of intensity control, talkers appeared to regulate loudness in response to the sound of their voices in their own ears, rather than to maintain intelligible communication (Garber, Siegel, and Pick, 1980; Haskell and Baken, 1978).

Finally, the effect of voice disorders on judgments of a talker's personality and appearance were investigated. Hypernasality evoked more negative evaluations than a harsh-breathy voice, but both were judged negatively in comparison with normal voices (Blood, Mahan, and Hyman, 1979).

TREATMENT

The published literature on treatment of voice disorders has been divided into three general topics. Under *voice therapy* are the articles dealing with the nature of this treatment process, its application, and results. Medical and surgical procedures deemed of interest to the speech pathologist are included under *laryngeal pathology*. *Spastic dysphonia* is discussed within a separate section for two reasons. First, it is the one clinical entity that has attracted considerable attention, but more important, the presumption of etiology that would be implied by inclusion under either of the other headings was conveniently avoided.

To increase credibility of the recent advances reported, the articles included in this chapter were subject to critical review, either by virtue of being published in refereed journals, or as papers presented as proceedings of scientific conferences. This criterion did not significantly exclude much work on assessment, but the bulk of nonmedical voice treatment procedures are not reported in journals. A major reason is that in recent years, criteria for publication of any therapy includes evidence of effectiveness. Reed (1980) has argued persuasively that as matters stand, the voice clinician must rely on opinions expressed in textbooks of authors who use different terms to describe different procedures based on different philosophies. He concludes that there is little scientific evidence that therapy techniques actually reduce vocal abuse.

Voice Therapy

Some considerations in approaching treatment of voice disorders have been reported since 1976. One was an acoustic method of evaluating voice improvement. Using a battery of acoustic measures, some (such as pitch and amplitude perturbation) correlated well with a trained listener's judgments of improvement in voice quality (Davis, 1982). Mysak (1977) has proposed a systems approach to voice disorders that casts the clinical problem in broad perspective of receptor, transmitter, facilitator, integrator, effector, and sensor systems. Brodnitz (1981), drawing on his wealth of experience, reminds the clinician that no amount of scientific progress will supplant the necessity of addressing the psychologic aspects of patients with voice disorders.

Two studies demonstrated that vocal performance can be changed with behavioral shaping procedures, and a footnote was added in another report warning of the hazards to health of using peanuts as reinforcers (Drudge and Philips, 1976; Lodge and Yarnall, 1981; Putnam, 1981).

Two cases, one treated with vocal rest, the other with a "pushing" technique, were reported. The traumatic effects on family, friends, and professional life of prolonged vocal rest following surgical removal of a nodule are described by the patient, a speech pathologist. As a consequence, she has sworn off complete vocal rest as routine therapy for patients recovering from laryngeal surgery (Fiedler, 1977). In the other case, a "hysterical" high pitch was lowered by obtaining low grunting sounds while the patient pulled herself down into her chair. Control and use of these pitched sounds were then extended (Aldes, 1981).

Therapy of vocal hyperfunction, the problem most frequently requiring intervention by voice clinicians, was the subject of only two investigations, both involving biofeedback. In one, EMG biofeedback from surface electrodes over the cricothyroid region was provided to six subjects with vocal hyperfunction. The three who had a normal larynx reduced EMG activity during speech and were judged to show improvement in quality. The other three, with spastic dysphonia or laryngeal lesions, did not improve (Prosek, Montgomery, Walden, and Schwartz, 1978). In the other study, five of seven improved (Stemple, Weiler, Whitehead, and Komray, 1980).

The full potential of biofeedback techniques will probably not be reached until far more is known about muscular activity during hyperfunction and optimal vocal function. Clearly, all laryngeal muscles do not relax during efficient phonation. With surface electrodes, biofeedback presently does not distinguish between those muscles that should relax and those that should contract.

Laryngeal Pathology

The primary purpose of phonosurgery is to improve voice. It takes five forms: extirpation of a lesion, laryngeal framework surgery to indirectly alter cord shape or mobility, direct cord surgery, neurosurgery to remobilize a paralyzed cord, and laryngeal reconstruction. The mechanisms of hoarseness, breathiness, roughness, and normal voice have been experimentally demonstrated to involve interactions among tightness of glottal closure, cord stiffness, and subglottal pressure. With closure too tight or pressure too high, roughness results. With incomplete cord closure, breathiness is heard (Isshiki, 1980).

Advances in phonosurgery since 1976 (other than for spastic dysphonia) have been mainly concerned with treatment of unilateral laryngeal paralysis. Isolated reports of management of other pathologies affecting voice range from procedures for papilloma to contact ulcers.

Laryngeal Paralysis

According to Tucker (1980), the most successful clinical strategy for unilateral laryngeal paralysis is patience. Out of 210 cases, 64 per cent recovered without therapy. Of the remainder, 26 per cent were helped with Teflon injections into the paralyzed cord to bring it into better approximation with the healthy cord. Similar success with Teflon has been reported by others (Reich and Lerman, 1978). Lewy (1976), who reviewed his results with 218 patients and reports on 1139 other cases, concluded that most persons recover voice. In a review of the literature, Montgomery (1979) indicated that when treatment is successful, the permanent level of improvement is reached in two to four weeks. A surgical correction for one of those causes of failure, excessive injection of Teflon, has also been devised (Horn and Dedo, 1980).

Two alternatives to vocal cord injection have been used to improve voice in cases of unilateral paralysis. (In bilateral paralysis, caused in over half of cases by thyroid surgery, restoration of the airway is the overriding concern. Preservation of whatever voice is possible is secondary; hence, the procedures are not classified as phonosurgery.) One is reinnervation of the paralyzed cord. Despite numerous earlier unsuccessful attempts, recent developments have provided some improvement in cases where the glottal chink was too great for vocal cord injection to be used (Isshiki, 1980; Sato and Ogura, 1978; Tucker, 1977, 1980). The other alternative that has produced dramatically improved voice in the few cases in which it has been used is to adduct the immobile arytenoid by applying tension to sutures, which simulates contraction of the paralyzed lateral cricoarytenoid muscle (Baken and Isshiki, 1977; Isshiki, 1977b; Isshiki, Tanabe, and Sawada, 1978).

Phonosurgery

Two procedures that have made phonosurgery possible are microlaryngeal techniques and laser surgery. With binocular microscope and stroboscopic illumination, the surgeon can make judgments on the basis of the vibratory pattern of the vocal cords. Preservation of mobility of the mucosa of the cords is especially important to prevention of hoarseness. Mucosal suppleness can be detected only when the cords vibrate, so the ability to observe them vibrating during surgery is a significant achievement in preservation of voice. The other procedure, laser surgery, often performed by use of the operating microscope, provides precision, safety, and prompt healing with minimal scarring when applied to small lesions such as nodules, polyps, papilloma, and cysts (Dedo and Izdebski, 1978; Isshiki, 1980).

The need to raise or lower pitch may arise from numerous conditions, not the least of which is transsexual operations. One condition that has been studied is the considerably higher fundamental frequency that follows treatment of asthma with prolonged administration of triamcinolone acetonide (Watkin and Ewanowski, 1979). Several experimental phonosurgical procedures have been used to change pitch. To raise it, cricothyroid approximation with sutures has been used to lengthen and thin the vocal folds. Also, injections of steroids to induce atrophy, and longitudinal incisions of the cords to weaken their resistance to elongation, have been attempted with limited success. To lower pitch, mass has been increased with vocal cord injections, neural supply to the cricothyroid muscle has been sectioned, and thyroplasty has been used in which portions of the thyroid cartilage were removed to shorten the cords. Although success is possible, these are procedures of last resort (Isshiki, 1980).

Other therapies of such lesions have also been reported. Skin grafts were used in 26 adults with papilloma; there was no recurrence in the transplant areas and voice was improved in 21 of the cases (Neumann and Ahmed, 1978). Medication was effective in relief of contact ulcers and granulomas caused by acid regurgitation secondary to hiatal hernia. For the mechanical causes of this functional pathology, which are usually habitual throat clearing and excessive glottal attacks, voice therapy was of value (Ward, Zwitman, Hanson, and Berci, 1980). To avoid the stiff mucosal scar, which impairs vibration, the traditional stripping of polypoid swelling was replaced with a sucking technique. Although this technique preserved the mucosal cord edge, voice improvement was not significantly better than with stripping (Hirano et al., 1981).

Spastic Dysphonia

Since the advent of surgical section of the recurrent laryngeal nerve as a treatment of spastic dysphonia, the procedure has been replicated with considerable success (Barton, 1979; Dedo, 1976, 1977; Levine, Wood, Batza, Rusnov, and Tucker, 1979). Similar improvement has been reported with modifications of the procedure, laryngeal nerve crush (a crushed nerve will regenerate, a sectioned nerve will not) being one example and selective section another. Selective section of the adductor, but not the abductor, branch of the recurrent nerve was attempted to preserve abduction during inspiration while retaining relief from hyperadduction during phonation (Biller, Som, and Lawson, 1979; Carpenter, Henley-Cohn, and Snyder, 1979; Lawrence, 1979).

At a symposium in 1979, these new surgical techniques and their results were discussed. All participants agreed that the cause of spastic dysphonia was unknown but that recurrent nerve section is the best treatment available. The typical result following surgery is relief from strain, but with an accompanying breathy, weak voice. Some reported that by the use of nerve crush, full voice returns when the nerve regenerates. Dedo attempted the same procedure, but spasticity returned along with nerve function. Iwamura described a technique in which selective section was done internally in the larynx instead of by the typical external procedure. Followup speech therapy was critical to his success. It apparently was also essential to Dedo's recurrent section procedure. DeSanto traced the results of sectioning in 27 patients whose voices were free of strain following surgery. Without further therapy, most improved for one month, then stayed the same. A few continued to improve, and 14 became worse (Lawrence, 1979).

The idea of intentionally inducing unilateral laryngeal paralysis, the consequence of recurrent nerve section, is troubling to many laryngologists. Although a case in which a sectioned recurrent nerve did regenerate has been reported, it is a rare exception (Wilson, Oldring, and Mueller, 1980). The predictable outcome is permanent paralysis with cord atrophy within a month. Although spasticity returns in 10 to 15 per cent of patients whose recurrent nerves are sectioned, it apparently results from development of compensatory attempts to achieve loudness (Dedo and Shipp, 1980). In one case, however, it resulted from reinnervation of the sectioned nerve.

The predictable outcome of recurrent nerve section is permanent paralysis. This traumatic outcome, coupled with the lurking suspicion that spastic dysphonia can result from many causes, including functional ones, impels a continuing search for less traumatic treatment (Isshiki, 1980; Lawrence, 1979). Still, it works well with some, and temporary chemical paralysis prior to surgery provides a reasonably accurate preview of the postsurgical voice (Izdebski, Shipp, and Dedo, 1979). Moreover, compensatory surgery is available to enlarge or thin the cord as necessary. Most important, voice therapy, designed along the lines of treatment of unilateral paralysis (which it is, indeed), is vital to optimize postsurgical vocal usage (Dedo and Shipp, 1980).

SUMMING UP

This review leaves no doubt that voice clinicians as well as voice scientists and laryngologists are searching for measures of laryngeal and vocal performance that are accurate and reliable. With them, communication among clinicians as well as scientists is enhanced. This objective is entirely commendable.

The picture that emerges is that virtually all of the recent advances have been in the detection and treatment of laryngeal pathology. Many of these advances have been accomplished by speech scientists and speech pathologists. They have played a dominant role in the development of noninvasive, acoustic, optic, behavioral, aerodynamic, and electromyographic methods of assessing laryngeal pathology. The importance of this contribution cannot be diminished.

What is notable by its absence is any attention to the causes or treatment of functional dysphonia. What has been studied are the *consequences* of vocal abuse. Especially useful have been the investigations of vocal fold reactions to stress. However, neither laryngologists nor voice clinicians or scientists have shown any research interest in *causes* of vocal abuse. Neither have they shown much interest in its treatment, 2 case studies of biofeedback effects on hyperfunction out of 170 research reports being the sum total. Spastic dysphonia and laryngeal paralysis have dominated the literature on assessment as well as on treatment since 1976.

A question that arises is what role speech pathologists seek in the management of voice disorders. Judging from this review, the only activity in which their publications show interest is assessment of vocal function, especially in laryngeal pathology. This view is reflected in the most sophisticated scientific work and also in activities of the clinic as reflected in the following argument for the speech pathologists's use of fiberoptics in indirect laryngoscopy: "There is a growing recognition that the role of voice clinician goes beyond that of technician. . . . Such evaluations enable the speech pathologist to ask the laryngologist specific and relevant questions concerning each case, to note the surgeon's success in restoring normal tissue contour, and to interpret the laryngologist's findings. Thus, the speech pathologist becomes a more dynamic, vital, and integral member of the team" (Chapey and Salzberg, 1981, pp. 87–88).

Granting that skill in visualizing the larynx has merit for voice clinicians, it is puzzling how this skill, or other assessment techniques, moves speech pathologists beyond the role of technician and gives them more vital functions on the team of voice specialists. Presumably, each specialist can make a unique contribution to the remediation of a voice problem, but it is not clear how voice clinicians differentiate their contribution from that of the laryngologist. The first professional judgment to be made in managing a voice disorder is the diagnosis of the nature and cause of the laryngeal condition. Physicians can enlist whatever technical input is necessary from such procedures as laryngoscopy, radiography, histology, and acoustic analyses, but by virtue of their training and licensing, they are solely qualified to make a diagnosis. The only role in which the voice clinician can function in the diagnostic process is to provide technical support. This can be an important role, but it does not define a contribution that the speech pathologist is better qualified to make than anyone else.

As for treatment, surgical or medical intervention is, of course, the exclusive province of physicians. One of the most frequent problems they encounter, however, is functional dysphonia, for which neither surgical nor medical relief is appropriate. If the speech pathologist has a unique contribution, it appears to be as a specialist in the nature, causes, and treatment of vocal abuse. Yet, this is the area in which virtually no investigation could be found for this review.

Why have voice scientists and clinicians investigated what are essentially the laryngologist's problems rather than the speech pathologist's? Suspected reasons are dimly visible. One is that descriptions of vocal behavior, abusive as well as normal, have been so nebulous as to preclude definition and measurement. Feedback control of voice is by ear and by feel. Neither sensation lends itself to unambiguous description. The concept of hyperfunction is as close as clinicians have come to a causal explanation of functional dysphonia. It is only a description, however, of the general feeling of tightness and strain in the throat. Because vibratory characteristics, to say nothing of patterns of muscular contraction, of any type of vocal production are unknown (hyperfunctional, abusive, efficient, or whatever), acoustic and physiologic measures of clinical importance have not been developed. Only perceptual descriptions are available, and even when clinicians and scientists are trained in their use, they do not permit acceptably valid and reliable communication. Probably the fundamental deterrent to scientific investigation of causes of functional dysphonia is the lack of accurate measures of clinically relevant vocal behavior.

For this reason, and possibly others, voice therapy has been passed along from generation to generation as a clinical art, complete with idiosyncratic perceptual descriptions dispensed by authorities in their texts. Rarely have any of the multitude of techniques recommended been tested for effectiveness and subjected to the scrutiny of peer review in scientific journals. This does not mean they are useless, but that we have no knowledge of what they accomplish, if they accomplish anything. As matters stand, we have little evidence by which to select with confidence those methods that are appropriate for any particular voice disorder. Until such evidence becomes available, the answer to Paul Moore's question, "Have the major issues in voice disorders been answered by speech science?", will remain "no."

REFERENCES

Aldes, M. (1981). Hysterical high pitch in an adult female: A case study. *Journal of Communication Disorders, 14,* 59-63.

Aminoff, M., Dedo, H., and Izdebski, K. (1978). Clinical aspects of spasmodic dysphonia. *Journal of Neurology, Neurosurgery, and Psychiatry, 41,* 361-365.

Andrews, A. Gould-Andrews fiberoptic laryngoscope. *(1977). In V. Lawrence (Ed.), Transcripts of the Sixth Symposium: Care of the professional voice.* New York: The Voice Foundation.

Aronson, A., and Hartman, D. (1981). Adductor spastic dysphonia as a sign of essential (voice) tremor. *Journal of Speech and Hearing Disorders, 46,* 52-58.

Askenfelt, A., Gauffin, J., Sundberg, J., and Kitzing, J. (1980). Vocal fundamental frequency as measured from contact microphone and electroglottograph recordings. A comparison of contact microphone and electroglottograph for the measurement of vocal fundamental frequency. *Journal of Speech and Hearing Research, 23,* 258-274.

Bacon, M., and Wolfe, V. (1980). Response to Zwitman. *Journal of Speech and Hearing Disorders, 45,* 568.

Baken, R., (1979). Respiratory mechanisms: Introduction and overview. In V. Lawrence (Ed.), *Transcripts of the Eighth Symposium: Care of the professional voice. Part II. Respiratory and phonatory control mechanisms.* New York: The Voice Foundation.

Baken, R., and Cavallo, S. (1979). Chest wall preparation for phonation in untrained speakers. In V. Lawrence (Ed.), *Transcripts of the Eighth Symposium: Care of the professional voice. Part II. Respiratory and Phonatory Control Mechanisms.* New York: The Voice Foundation.

Baken, R., and Cavallo, S. (1981). Prephonatory chest wall posturing. *Folia Phoniatrica, 33,* 193-203.

Baken, R., and Isshiki, N. (1977). Arytenoid displacement by simulated intrinsic muscle contraction. *Folia Phoniatrica, 29,* 206-216.

Barton, R. (1979). Treatment of spastic dysphonia by recurrent laryngeal nerve section. *Laryngoscope, 89,* 244-249.

Biller, H., Som, M., and Lawson, W. (1979). Laryngeal nerve crush for spasmodic dysphonia. *Annals of Otolaryngology, 88,* 531-532.

Blood, G., Mahan, G., and Hyman, M. (1979). Judging personality and appearance from voice disorders. *Journal of Communication Disorders, 12,* 63-67.

Bocchino, J., and Tucker, H. (1978). Recurrent laryngeal nerve pathology in spasmodic dysphonia. *Laryngoscope, 88,* 1274-1280.

Boone, D. (1983). Voice disorders in children and adults. *Seminars in Speech and Language, 4,* 189-286.

Bralley, R., Bull, J., Gore, C., and Edgerton, M. (1978). Evaluation of vocal pitch in male transsexuals. *Journal of Communication Disorders, 11,* 443-449.

Brindle, B., and Morris, H. (1979). Prevalence of voice quality deviations in the normal adult population. *Journal of Communication Disorders, 12,* 439–445.

Brodnitz, F. (1976). Spastic dysphonia. *Annals of Otology, Rhinology, and Laryngology, 85,* 210–214.

Brodnitz, F. (1978). Adolescent voice disorders. In B. Weinberg (Ed.), *Transcripts of the Seventh Symposium: Care of the professional voice. Part II: Life span changes in the human voice.* New York: The Voice Foundation.

Brodnitz, F. (1981). Psychological considerations in vocal rehabilitation. *Journal of Speech and Hearing Disorders, 46,* 21–16

Brown, W., and Feinstein, S. (1977). Speaker sex identification in Wilson's disease. *Folia Phoniatrica, 29,* 240–248.

Cannito, M., and Johnson, J. (1981). Spastic dysphonia: A continuum disorder. *Journal of Communication Disorders, 14,* 215–223.

Carpenter, R., Henley-Cohn, J., and Snyder, G. (1979). Spastic dysphonia: Treatment by selective section of the recurrent laryngeal nerve. *Laryngoscope, 89,* 2000–2003.

Chapey, R., and Salzberg, A. (1981). The speech clinician's use of fiberoptics in indirect laryngoscopy. *Journal of Communication Disorders, 14,* 87–90.

Childers, D., Paige, A., and Moore, G. (1976). Laryngeal vibration patterns: Machine-aided measurements from high-speed film. *Archives of Otolaryngology, 102,* 407–410.

Cohen, D., Shaywitz, B., Caparulo, B., Young, G., and Bowers, M. (1978). Chronic, multiple tics of Gilles de la Tourette's disease. *Archives of General Psychiatry, 35,* 245–250.

Coleman, R. (1976). A comparison of the contributions of two voice quality characteristics to the perception of maleness and femaleness in the voice. *Journal of Speech and Hearing Research, 19,* 168–180.

Coleman, R., Mabis, J., and Hinson, J. (1977). Fundamental frequency-sound pressure level profiles of adult male and female voices. *Journal of Speech and Hearing Research, 20,* 197–204.

Colton, R., and Estill, J. (1976). Perceptual differentiation of voice modes. In V. Lawrence (Ed.), *Transcripts of the Fifth Symposium: Care of the professional voice.* New York: The Voice Foundation.

Colton, R., and Estill, J. (1978). Mechanisms of voice quality variation: Voice modes. In V. Lawrence (Ed.), *Transcripts of the Seventh Symposium: Care of the professional voice. Part I: The scientific papers.* New York: The Voice Foundation.

Colton, R., Estill, J., and Gould, L. (1977). Physiology of voice modes: Vocal tract characteristics. In V. Lawrence (Ed.) *Transcripts of the Sixth Symposium: Care of the professional voice.* New York: The Voice Foundation.

Darby, J., and Hollien, H. (1977). Vocal and speech patterns of depressive patients. *Folia Phoniatrica, 29,* 279–241.

Davis, S. (1976). Computer evaluation of laryngeal pathology based on inverse filtering of speech. *SCRL Monograph, 13,* Santa Barbara, CA: Speech Communication Research Laboratory.

Davis, S. (1979). Acoustic characteristics of normal and pathological voices. In N. Lass (Ed.), *Speech and language: Research and theory.* New York: Academic Press.

Davis, S. (1982). Acoustic characteristics of normal and pathological voices. In Proceedings of the Conference on the Assessment of Vocal Pathology. *ASHA Reports, 11,* 97–115.

Dedo, H. (1976). Recurrent laryngeal nerve section for spastic dysphonia. *Annals of Otology, Rhinology, and Laryngology, 85,* 451–459.

Dedo, H. (1977). Surgical treatment of spastic dysphonia. In V. Lawrence (Ed.), *Transcripts of the Sixth Symposium: Care of the professional voice.* New York: The Voice Foundation.

Dedo, H., and Izdebski, K. (1978). The effects on voice upon removing certain vocal fold lesions. In V. Lawrence (Ed.), *Transcripts of the Seventh Symposium: Care of the professional voice. Part III: Medical/surgical therapy.* New York: The Voice Foundation.

Dedo, H., Izdebski, K., and Townsend, J. (1977). Recurrent laryngeal nerve histopathology in spastic dysphonia. *Annals of Otolaryngology, 86,* 806–812.

Dedo, H., and Shipp, T. (1980). *Spastic dysphonia: A surgical and voice therapy treatment program.* San Diego: College-Hill Press.

Dedo, H., Townsend, J., and Izdebski, K. (1978). Current evidence for the organic etiology of spastic dysphonia. *ORL, 86,* 875–880.

Dordain, M., and Chevrie-Muller, C. (1977). Voice and speech in Wilson's disease. *Folia Phoniatrica, 29,* 217–232.

Drudge, M., and Philips, B. (1976). Shaping behavior in voice therapy. *Journal of Speech and Hearing Disorders, 41,* 398–411.

Eckel, F., and Boone, D. (1981). The s/z ratio as an indicator of laryngeal pathology. *Journal of Speech and Hearing Disorders, 46,* 147–149.

Emanuel, F., and Austin, D. (1981). Identification of normal and abnormally rough vowels by spectral noise level measurements. *Journal of Communication Disorders, 14,* 75–85.

Emanuel, F., and Scarzini, A. (1979). Vocal register effects on vowel spectral noise and roughness: Findings for adult females. *Journal of Communication Disorders, 12,* 263–272.

Emanuel, F., and Scarzini, A. (1980). Vocal register effects on vowel spectral noise and roughness: Findings for adult males. *Journal of Communication Disorders, 13,* 121–131.

Fiedler, I. (1977). Vocal rest. *ASHA, 19,* 307–308.

Forner, L., and Hixon, T. (1977). Respiratory kinematics in profoundly hearing-impaired speakers. *Journal of Speech and Hearing Research, 20,* 373–408.

Fourcin, A. (1982). Laryngographic assessment of phonatory function. In Proceedings of the Conference on the Assessment of Vocal Pathology, *ASHA Reports, 11,* 116–127.

Fritzell, B., Hammarberg, B., and Wedin, L. (1977). Clinical applications of acoustic voice analysis, Part I. *Quarterly Progress and Status Report.* Stockholm: Speech Transmission Laboratory, Royal Institute of Technology.

Fujimura, O. (1982). Fiberoptic observation and measurement of vocal fold movement. In Proceedings of the Conference on the Assessment of Vocal Pathology. *ASHA Reports, 11,* 59–69.

Fujimura, O., Baer, T., and Niimi, S. (1979). A stereo-fiberscope with a magnetic interlens bridge for laryngeal observation. *Journal of the Acoustical Society of America, 65,* 478–480.

Garber, S., and Moller, K. (1979). The effects of feedback filtering on nasalization in normal and hypernasal speakers. *Journal of Speech and Hearing Research, 22,* 321–333.

Garber, S., Siegel, G., and Pick, H. (1980). The effects of feedback filtering on speaker intelligibility. *Journal of Communication Disorders, 13,* 289–294.

Gauffin, J., and Sundberg, J. (1977). Clinical applications of acoustic voice analysis, Part II. *Quarterly Progress and Status Report.* Stockholm: Speech Transmission Laboratory, Royal Institute of Technology.

Golden, G. (1977). Tourette syndrome. *American Journal of Diseases of Children, 131,* 531–534.

Gordon, M., Morton, F., and Simpson, I. (1978). Air flow measurements in diagnosis, assessment, and treatment of mechanical dysphonia. *Folia Phoniatrica, 30,* 166–174.

Gould, W. (1979). Interrelationship between voice and laryngeal mucosal reflexes. In V. Lawrence (Ed.), *Transcripts of the Eighth Symposium: Care of the professional voice. Part II. Respiratory and phonatory control mechanisms.* New York: The Voice Foundation.

Gould, W., Kojima, H., and Lambiase, A. (1979). A technique for stroboscopic examination of the vocal folds using fiberoptics. *Archives of Otolaryngology, 105,* 285.

Guidi, G., Bannister, R., Gibson, W., and Payne, J. (1981). Laryngeal electromyography in multiple system atrophy with autonomic failure. *Journal of Neurology, Neurosurgery and Psychiatry, 44,* 49–53.

Hall, J., and Jerger, J. (1976). Acoustic reflex characteristics in spastic dysphonia. *Archives of Otolaryngology, 102,* 411–415.

Hamlet, S. (1982). Ultra-sound assessment of phonatory function. In Proceedings of the *Conference on the Assessment of Vocal Pathology. ASHA Reports, 11,* 128–140.

Hamlet, S., Geoffrey, V., and Bartlett, D. (1976). Effect of a dental prosthesis on speaker-specific characteristics of voice. *Journal of Speech and Hearing Research, 19,* 639–650.

Hanley, T., Hanson, R., and Miller, A. (1978). Young adult and middle-aged voice. In B. Weinberg (Ed.), *Transcripts of the Seventh Symposium: Care of the professional voice, Part II: Life span changes in the human voice.* New York: The Voice Foundation.

Hanson, W., and Emanuel, F. (1979). Spectral noise and vocal roughness relationships in adults with laryngeal pathology. *Journal of Communication Disorders, 12,* 113–124.

Harris, K. (1982). Electromyography as a technique for laryngeal investigation. In Proceedings of the Conference on the Assessment of Vocal Pathology. *ASHA Reports, 11,* 70–87.

Hartman, D. (1979). The perceptual identity and characteristics of aging in normal male adult speakers. *Journal of Speech and Hearing Disorders, 12,* 53–61.

Hartman, D., and Aronson, A. (1981). Clinical investigations of intermittent breathy dysphonia. *Journal of Speech and Hearing Disorders, 46,* 428–432.

Hasek, C., Singh, S., and Murry, T. (1980). Acoustic attributes of pre-adolescent voices. *Journal of the Acoustical Society of America, 68,* 1262–1265.

Haskell, J., and Baken, R. (1978). Self perception of speaking pitch levels. *Journal of Speech and Hearing Disorders, 43,* 3–8.

Hiki, S., Imazzumi, S., Hirano, M., Matsushita, H., and Kakita, Y. (1976). Acoustical analysis for voice disorders. *Conference Record, 1976 IEEE International Conference on Acoustics, Speech, and Signal Processing.* Rome, NY: Canterbury Press.

Hirano, M., Hiki, S., Imazzumi, S., Kakita, Y., and Matsushita, H. (1978). Acoustical analysis of pathological voice. In V. Lawrence (Ed.), *Transcripts of the Seventh Symposium: Care of the professional voice. Part III: Medical/surgical therapy.* New York: The Voice Foundation.

Hirano, M., Kurita, S., Matsuo, K., and Nagata, K. (1980). Laryngeal tissue reaction to stress. In V. Lawrence and B. Weinberg (Eds.), *Transcripts of the Ninth Symposium: Care of the professional voice. Part I: Physical factors, vocal function and control.* New York: The Voice Foundation.

Hirano, M., Kurita, S., Matsuo, K., and Nagata, K. (1981). Vocal fold polyp and polypoid vocal fold (Reinike's edema). *Journal of Research in Singing, 4,* 33–44.

Hirose, H., Sawashima, M., Ushijima, T., and Kumamoto, Y. (1977). Eunuchoidism: Voice pitch abnormality as an autonomous syndrome. *Folia Phoniatrica, 29,* 261–269.

Hixon, T., Mead, J., and Goldman, M. (1976). Dynamics of the chest wall during speech production: Function of the thorax, rib cage, diaphragm, and abdomen. *Journal of Speech and Hearing Research, 19,* 297–356.

Hollien, H. (1978). Adolescence and voice change. In B. Weinberg (Ed.), *Transcripts of the Seventh Symposium: Care of the professional voice. Part II: Life span changes in the human voice.* New York: The Voice Foundation.

Hollien, H., and Tolhurst, G. (1978). The aging voice. In B. Weinberg (Ed.), *Transcripts of the Seventh Symposium: Care of the professional voice. Part II: Life span changes in the human voice.* New York: The Voice Foundation.

Honjo, I., and Isshiki, M. (1980). Laryngoscopic and voice characteristics of aged persons. *Archives of Otolaryngology, 106,* 149-150.

Horii, Y. (1979). Fundamental frequency perturbation observed in sustained phonation. *Journal of Speech and Hearing Research, 22,* 5-19.

Horii, Y., and Ryan, W. (1981). Fundamental frequency characteristics and perceived age of adult male speakers. *Folia Phoniatrica, 33,* 227-233.

Horii, Y., and Weinberg, B. (1979). Sensory contributions to the control of phonation. In V. Lawrence (Ed.), *Transcripts of the Eighth Symposium: Care of the professional voice. Part II. Respiratory and phonatory control mechanisms.* New York: The Voice Foundation.

Horn, K., and Dedo, H. (1980). Surgical correction of the convex vocal cord after teflon injection. *Laryngoscope, 90,* 281-286.

Ishizaka, K., and Isshiki, N. (1976). Computer simulation of pathological vocal-cord vibration. *Journal of the Acoustical Society of America, 60,* 1193-1198.

Isshiki, N. (1977a). Clinical implication of computer simulation of false voice. In V. Lawrence (Ed.), *Transcripts of the Sixth Symposium: Care of the professional voice.* New York: The Voice Foundation.

Isshiki, N. (1977b). Functional surgery of the larynx. In V. Lawrence (Ed.), *Transcripts of the Sixth Symposium: Care of the professional voice.* New York: The Voice Foundation.

Isshiki, N., (1980). Recent advances in phonosurgery. *Folia Phoniatrica, 32,* 119-154.

Isshiki, N., Tanabe, M., Ishizaka, K., and Broad, C. (1977). Clinical significance of asymmetrical tension of the vocal cords. *Annals of Otology, Rhinology, and Laryngology, 86,* 1-9.

Isshiki, N., Tanabe, M., and Sawada, M. (1978). Arytenoid adduction for unilateral vocal cord paralysis. *Archives of Otolaryngology, 104,* 555-558.

Izdebski, K. (1977). Some data on spastic dysphonia patients. In V. Lawrence (Ed.), *Transcripts of the Sixth Symposium: Care of the professional voice.* New York: The Voice Foundation.

Izdebski, K., and Shipp, T. (1978). Minimal reaction times for phonatory initiation. *Journal of Speech and Hearing Research, 21,* 638-651.

Izdebski, K., Shipp, T., and Dedo, H. (1979). Predicting postoperative voice characteristics of spastic dysphonia patients. *Otolaryngology Head and Neck Surgery, 87,* 428-434.

Janfaza, P. (1978). New magnifying laryngeal and nasalpharyngeal mirrors. *Archives of Otolaryngology, 104,* 740.

Kahane, J. (1980). Age related histological changes in the human male and female laryngeal cartilages: Biological and functional implications. In V. Lawrence and B. Weinberg (Eds.), *Transcripts of the Ninth Symposium: Care of the professional voice. Part I. Physical factors, vocal function and control.* New York: The Voice Foundation.

Kelman, A., Gordon, M., Morton, F., and Simpson, I. (1981). Comparison of methods for assessing vocal function. *Folia Phoniatrica, 33,* 51-65.

Kitajima, K. (1981). Quantitative evaluation of the noise level in the pathologic voice. *Folia Phoniatrica, 33,* 115-124.

Kitajima, K., and Gould, W. (1976). Vocal shimmer in sustained phonation of normal and pathologic voice. *Annals of Otology, Rhinology, and Laryngology, 85,* 377-381.

Koike, K., Takahashi, H., and Calcaterra, T. (1977). Acoustic measures for detecing laryngeal pathology. *Acta Otolaryngologica, 84,* 105-117.

Lawrence, V. (1979). *Spastic dysphonia: State of the art 1979.* New York: The Voice Foundation.

Leonard, R., and Ringel, R. (1979). Vocal shadowing under conditions of normal and altered laryngeal sensation. *Journal of Speech and Hearing Research, 22,* 794-817.

Levine, H., Wood, B., Batza, E., Rusnov, M., and Tucker, H. (1979). Recurrent laryngeal nerve section for spasmodic dysphonia. *Annals of Otology, Rhinology, and Laryngology, 88,* 527–530.

Lewy, R. (1976). Experience with vocal cord injection. *Annals of Otology, Rhinology, and Laryngology, 85,* 440–450.

Lindblom, B., Lubker, J., and Pauli, S. (1977). An acoustic-perceptual method for the quantitative evaluation of hypernasality. *Journal of Speech and Hearing Research, 20,* 485–496.

Lodge, J., and Yarnall, G. (1981). A case study of vocal volume reduction. Journal of Speech and Hearing Disorders, 46, 317–320.

Logemann, J., Fisher, H., Boshes, B., and Blonsky, E. (1978). Frequency and co-occurrence of vocal tract dysfunctions in the speech of a large sample of Parkinson patients. *Journal of Speech and Hearing Disorders, 43,* 47–57.

Ludlow, C. (1982). Research needs for the assessment of phonatory function. In Proceedings of the Conference on the Assessment of Vocal Pathology. *ASHA Reports, 11,* 3–8.

Ludlow, C., and Bassich, C. (1981). The differential diagnosis of syndromes of dysarthria using measures of speech production. In N. Lass (Ed.), *Speech and language: Advances in basic research and practice.* Academic Press.

Ludlow, C., and Hart, M. (1982). Preface. Proceedings of the Conference on the Assessment of Vocal Pathology. *ASHA Reports, 11,* v.

Markel, J., and Gray, A. (1976). *Linear prediction of speech.* New York: Springer-Verlag.

McCall, G. (1977). Studies in spastic dysphonia: Projected research concerned with central neurologic pathologies on laryngeal dysfunction. In V. Lawrence (Ed.), *Transcripts of the Sixth Symposium: Care of the professional voice.* New York: The Voice Foundation.

Merson, R., and Ginsberg, A. (1979). Spasmodic dysphonia: Abductor type. A clinical report of acoustic, aerodynamic, and perceptual characteristics. *Laryngoscope, 89,* 129–139.

Monsen, R. (1982). The use of the reflectionless tube to assess vocal function. In Proceedings of the Conference on the Assessment of Vocal Pathology. *ASHA Reports, 11,* 141–150.

Montgomery, W. (1979). Laryngeal paralysis: Teflon injection. *Annals of Otology, Rhinology, and Laryngology, 88,* 647–657.

Moore, G. (1976). Observations of laryngeal disease, laryngeal behavior and voice. *Annals of Otology, Rhinology, and Laryngology, 85,* 553–565.

Moore, P. (1977). Have the major issues in voice disorders been answered by research in speech science? A 50-year retrospective. *Journal of Speech and Hearing Disorders, 42,* 152–160.

Murry, T. (1978). Speaking fundamental frequency characteristics associated with voice pathologies. *Journal of Speech and Hearing Disorders, 43,* 374–379.

Murry, T., and Doherty, E. (1980). Selected acoustic characteristics of pathologic and normal speakers. *Journal of Speech and Hearing Research, 23,* 361–369.

Murry, T., and Singh, S. (1980). Multidimensional analysis of male and female voices. *Journal of the Acoustical Society of America, 68,* 1294–1300.

Murry, T., Singh, S., and Sargent, M. (1977). Multidimensional classification of abnormal voice qualities. *The Journal of the Acoustical Society of America, 61,* 1630–1635.

Mysak, E. (1977). Systems approach to voice disorders. In V. Lawrence (Ed.), *Transcripts of the Sixth Symposium: Care of the professional voice.* New York: The Voice Foundation.

Neumann, O., and Ahmed, M. (1978). A new approach to the treatment of laryngeal papilloma in adults. *Journal of Laryngology and Otology, 92,* 325–331.

Nichols, A. (1979). Jitter and shimmer related to vocal roughness. *Journal of Speech and Hearing Research, 22,* 670–671.

Parnes, S., Lavarato, A., and Myers, E. (1978). Study of spastic dysphonia using fiberoptic laryngoscopy. *Annals of Otology, Rhinology, and Laryngology, 87,* 322-326.

Pederson, M. (1977). Electroglottography compared with synchronized stroboscopy in normal persons. *Folia Phoniatrica, 29,* 191-199.

Perkins, W. (1978). Mechanisms of vocal abuse. In B. Weinberg (Ed.), *Transcripts of the Seventh Symposium: Care of the professional voice. Part II: Life span changes in the human voice.* New York: The Voice Foundation.

Portnoy, R. (1979). Hyperkinetic dysarthria as an early indicator of impending tardive dyskinesia. *Journal of Speech and Hearing Disorders, 44,* 214-219.

Proctor, D. (1979). Breath, the power source for the voice. In V. Lawrence (Ed.), *Transcripts of the Eighth Symposium: Care of the professional voice. Part II. Respiratory and phonatory control mechanisms.* New York: The Voice Foundation.

Prosek, R., Montgomery, A., Walden, B., and Schwartz, D. (1978). EMG biofeedback in the treatment of hyperfunctional voice disorders. *Journal of Speech and Hearing Disorders, 43,* 282-294.

Putnam, A. (1981). Caution. . .peanuts may be harmful to your clients' health. *Journal of Speech and Hearing Disorders, 46,* 220-221.

Ravits, J., Aronson, A., DeSanto, L., and Dyck, P. (1979). No morphometric abnormality of recurrent laryngeal nerve in spastic dysphonia. *Neurology, 29,* 1376-1382.

Reed, C. (1980). Voice therapy: A need for research. *Journal of Speech and Hearing Disorders, 45,* 157-169.

Reich, A., and Lerman, J. (1978). Teflon laryngoplasty: An acoustical and perceptual case study. *Journal of Speech and Hearing Research, 43,* 496-505.

Rothenberg, M. (1977). Measurement of air flow in speech. *Journal of Speech and Hearing Research, 20,* 155-176.

Rothenberg, M. (1982). Some relations between glottal air flow and vocal fold contact area. In Proceedings of the Conference on the Assessment of Vocal Pathology. *ASHA Reports, 11,* 88-96.

Saito, S., Fukuda, H., Kitahara, S., and Kokawa, N. (1978). Stroboscopic observation of vocal fold vibration with fiberoptics. *Folia Phoniatrica, 30,* 241-244.

Sato, F., and Ogura, J. (1978). Functional restoration for recurrent laryngeal nerve paralysis: an experimental study. *Laryngoscope, 88,* 855-871.

Sawashima, M. (1976). Fiberoptic observation of the larynx and other speech organs. In M. Sawashima and F. Cooper, (Eds.), *Dynamic aspects of speech production.* Tokyo: University of Tokyo Press.

Schiff, M. (1977). Medical management of acute laryngitis. In V. Lawrence (Ed.), *Transcripts of the Sixth Symposium: Care of the professional voice.* New York: The Voice Foundation.

Schiff, M., and Gould, W. (1978). Hormones and their influence on the performer's voice. In V. Lawrence (Ed.), *Transcripts of the Seventh Symposium: Care of the professional voice. Part III: Medical/surgical therapy.* New York: The Voice Foundation.

Schultz-Coulon, H., Battmer, R., and Reichers, H. (1979). The 3-kHz formant-a criterion for the evaluation of vocal efficiency? I. The untrained normal voice. II. The trained singing voice. *Folia Phoniatrica, 31,* 291-313.

Sharbrough, F., Stockard, J., and Aronson, A. (1978). Brainstem auditory evoked responses in spastic dysphonia. *Transactions of American Neurology, 103,* 198-201.

Shipp, T., Mueller, P., and Zwitman, D. (1980). Intermittent abductory dysphonia. *Journal of Speech and Hearing Disorders, 45,* 283.

Silverman, E., and Zimmer, C. (1978). Effect of the menstrual cycle on voice quality. *Archives of Otolaryngology, 104,* 7-10.

Singh, S., and Murry, T. (1978). Multidimensional classification of normal voice qualities. *Journal of the Acoustical Society of America, 64,* 81–87.

Smitheran, J., and Hixon, T. (1981). A clinical method for estimating laryngeal airway resistance during vowel production. *Journal of Speech and Hearing Disorders, 46,* 138–146.

Sorenson, D., Horii, Y., and Leonard, R. (1980). Effects of laryngeal topical anesthesia on voice fundamental frequency perturbation. *Journal of Speech and Hearing Research, 23,* 274–283.

Stemple, J., Weiler, E., Whitehead, W., and Komray, R. (1980). Electromyographic biofeedback training with patients exhibiting a hyperfunctional voice disorder. *Laryngoscope, 90,* 471–476.

Stevens, K., and Hirano, M. (Eds.) (1980). *Vocal fold physiology.* Tokyo: University of Tokyo Press.

Stevens, K., Nickersen, R., Boothroyd, A., and Rollins, A. (1976). Assessment of nasalization in the speech of deaf children. *Journal of Speech and Hearing Research, 19,* 393–416.

Stoicheff, M. (1981). Speaking fundamental frequency characteristics of nonsmoking female adults. *Journal of Speech and Hearing Research, 24,* 437–441.

Sweeting, P. (1979). Voice onset time and vowel duration in the normal aged population: Implications for phonatory control. In V. Lawrence (Ed.), *Transcripts of the Eighth Symposium: Care of the professional voice. Part II. Respiratory and phonatory control mechanisms.* New York: The Voice Foundation.

Teany, D. (1980). The electroglottograph as a clinical tool for the observation and analysis of vocal fold vibration. In V. Lawrence and B. Weinberg (Eds.), *Transcripts of the Ninth Symposium: Care of the professional voice. Part II: Vocal stress—Medical diagnosis/treatment.* New York: The Voice Foundation.

Todt, E., and Howell, R. (1980). Vocal cues as indices of schizophrenia. *Journal of Speech and Hearing Research, 23,* 517–526.

Tucker, H. (1977). Reinnervation of the unilaterally paralyzed larynx. *Annals of Otology, Rhinology, and Laryngology, 86,* 789–794.

Tucker, H. (1980). Vocal cord paralysis—etiology and management. *Laryngoscope, 90,* 585–590.

Tuomi, S., and Fisher, J. (1979). Characteristics of simulated sexy voice. *Folia Phoniatrica, 31,* 242–249.

Ward, P., Hanafee, W., Mancuso, A., Shallit, J., and Berci, G. (1979). Evaluation of computerized tomography, cinelaryngoscopy, and laryngography in determining the extent of laryngeal disease. *Annals of Otology, Rhinology, and Laryngology, 88,* 454–462.

Ward, P., Zwitman, D., Hanson, D., and Berci, G. (1980). Contact ulcers and granulomas of the larynx: New insights into their etiology as a basis for more rational treatment. *Otolaryngology and Head and Neck Surgery, 88,* 262–269.

Watkin, K., and Ewanowski, S. (1979). The effects of triamcinolone acetonide on the voice. *Journal of Speech and Hearing Research, 22,* 446–455.

Weinberg, G. (1978). Evolution/involution of the human voice summary with an introduction to age-associated voice disorders. In B. Weinberg (Ed.), *Transcripts of the Seventh Symposium: Care of the professional voice. Part II: Life span changes in the human voice.* New York: The Voice Foundation.

Wendler, J., Doherty, E., and Hollien, H. (1980). Voice classification by means of long-term speech spectra. *Folia Phoniatrica, 32,* 51–60.

Whitehead, R., and Lieberth, A. (1979). Spectrographic and perceptual features of vocal tension/harshness in hearing impaired adults. *Journal of Communication Disorders, 12,* 83–92.

Wilder, C. (1980). Vocal aging. In B. Weinberg (Ed.), *Transcripts of the Seventh Symposium: Care of the professional voice. Part II: Life span changes in the human voice.* New York: The Voice Foundation.

Wilder, C. (1979). Chest wall preparation for phonation in untrained speakers. In V. Lawrence (Ed.), *Transcripts of the Eighth Symposium: Care of the professional voice. Part II. Respiratory and phonatory control mechanisms.* New York: The Voice Foundation.

Williams A., Hanson, D., and Calne, D. (1979). Vocal cord paralysis in the Shy-Drager syndrome. *Journal of Neurosurgery and Psychiatry, 42,* 151–153.

Wilson, F., Oldring, D., and Mueller, K. (1980). Recurrent laryngeal nerve dissection: A case report involving return of spastic dysphonia after initial surgery. *Journal of Speech and Hearing Disorders, 45,* 112–118.

Wirz, S., Subtelny, J., and Whitehead, R. (1981). Perceptual and spectrographic study of tense voice in normal hearing and deaf subjects. *Folia Phoniatrica, 33,* 23–36.

Wolfe, V., and Bacon, M. (1976). Spectrographic comparison of two types of spastic dysphonia. *Journal of Speech and Hearing Disorders, 41,* 325–332.

Wyke, B. (1979). Neurological aspects of phonatory control systems in the larynx: A review of current concepts. In V. Lawrence (Ed.), *Transcripts of the Eighth Symposium: Care of the professional voice. Part II. Respiratory and phonatory control mechanisms.* New York: The Voice Foundation.

Zwitman, D. (1979). Bilateral cord dysfunctions: Abductor type spastic dysphonia. *Journal of Speech and Hearing Disorders, 44,* 373–378.

Chapter 5

Speech Rehabilitation of the Laryngectomized Patient: Advances and Issues

Bernd Weinberg

An obvious and primary postsurgical rehabilitation objective for laryngectomized patients is the restoration of oral communication. Until recently, speech rehabilitation of laryngectomized patients has been accomplished chiefly with the time honored methods of esophageal speech or through the use of artificial larynges.

Unfortunately, major advances or improvements have not been made in the design of artificial larynges, and only slight improvements have been achieved in treatment for persons who use commercially available, artificial larynges. Although it is true that many laryngectomized patients are able to produce highly intelligible and functionally serviceable speech using these devices, studies dealing with important aspects of their use are scarce. The vocal output of users of artificial larynges is characterized by a non-normal, mechanical, or electronic quality with limited variation in f_0 (pitch) or intensity (loudness). Given the state of technology, efforts should be made to design more efficient voicing sources to provide laryngectomized patients with more normal sounding vocal attributes.

The use of speech and vocal synthesis in the commercial sector has proliferated at an accelerating rate. For example, witness the extent to which people interact with large numbers of "voices" in a vast array of toys, business transactions, and so on. Undoubtedly, the quality of "voices" used in these commercial applications will improve to the extent that many people may not realize that they are interacting with nonhuman devices. It would be a sad commentary on our social system and values if, a decade from now, people interacted with a host of natural sounding, synthetic sources, while human talkers deprived of a normal voicing source, yet richly

This chapter was prepared, in part, through support from an NIH Grant (Linguistic Aspects of Speech After Laryngectomy).

endowed with normal linguistic performance and competence, continued to produce speech characterized by significant liability or absence of natural quality.

In recent years, a steady flow of information has resulted in improved understanding of esophageal speech production (see Weinberg, 1980, for a review). Although basic attributes of esophageal speech production are now more clearly understood, significant numbers of laryngectomized patients fail to develop functionally serviceable speech despite having been exposed to adequate therapy. Hence, advances in assessment and therapy for persons seeking to use esophageal speech produced on a conventional basis as a primary form of oral communication have been limited. The recent observations that some alaryngeal talkers are able to realize prosodic features and linguistic contrasts does represent an important advance in current understanding (Gandour and Weinberg, 1982, 1983; Gandour, Weinberg, and Garzione, 1983; Gandour, Weinberg, and Kosowski, 1983; McHenry, Reich, and Minifie, 1982; Scarpino and Weinberg, 1981). These recent observations have important clinical and basic scientific implications. For example, it now appears inappropriate to assume that talkers using some major forms of alaryngeal speech are unable to approximate normal linguistic-prosodic patterns (e.g., stress, intonation, juncture). The observation that some alaryngeal talkers are able to realize prosodic patterns suggests that such patients have the capacity to produce speech at proficiency levels exceeding those typically searched for by professional workers in the field.

Undoubtedly, the more striking advances in the field of speech rehabilitation for laryngectomized patients are those associated with techniques currently being advocated for surgical-prosthetic management. The major focus of this chapter will be to review the advances made and to examine some questions occasioned by these developments.

SURGICAL PROSTHETIC APPROACHES TO SPEECH REHABILITATION

The more significant advances in the field of speech rehabilitation for laryngectomized patients are those related to surgical-prosthetic management. In the past decade, surgical-prosthetic approaches to speech restoration for laryngectomized patients have proliferated. Reviews of this recent proliferation are available in other sources (Shedd and Weinberg, 1980; Weinberg, 1980). The most significant contemporary advances in this field of endeavor relate to techniques and procedures advocated and used in conjunction with tracheoesophageal puncture (TEP) technique.

In 1980, Singer and Blom formally described an endoscopic technique for restoration after total laryngectomy. A comparable approach has been described by Panje (1981).

TECHNIQUE OUTCOMES: SPEECH RESULTS

The tracheoesophageal puncture approach to speech restoration for laryngectomized patients clearly represents a significant advance. At the time of this writing, carefully controlled studies have not been completed that enable us to specify the speech characteristics or levels of speech proficiency attained by patients undergoing this procedure. Informal descriptions of these attributes and levels have been published. For example, Singer and Blom (1980) initially described a two year, 60 patient experience with this method. Of the 60 patients, 54 (90 per cent) achieved what Singer and Blom refer to as "fluent voices and were satisfied with their communication ability" (p. 531). These patients achieved "satisfactory communication. . .regarded as intelligible and fluent to listeners" (p. 531). Conversely, the remaining six speakers (10 per cent) were classified as "nonfluent speakers or voice failures" (p. 531). In a more recent report, Singer, Blom, and Haymaker (1981) summarized their 40 month experience with 129 patients. Again using informal description, they indicated that "successful acquisition of voice occurred in 113 of the 129 patients (88%)" (p. 498).

The results of rehabilitation using the Singer-Blom method have also been described by others. For example, Wood, Rusnov, Tucker, and Levine (1981) recently summarized the results of experiences at the Cleveland Clinic with 30 total laryngectomy patients who underwent tracheoesophageal puncture. This group of clinicians categorized rehabilitation as successful "if the post-TEP [tracheoesophageal puncture] voice was judged better than the pre-TEP mode of communication by the patient, one or more family members, and the speech pathologist" (p. 493). On this basis 28 patients (93 per cent) were classified as successes, while two were regarded as failures.

Additional, independent descriptions of experiences with tracheoesophageal puncture have been offered by Wetmore, Johns, and Baker (1981). Their experiences reflect a multi-institutional (University of Virginia, University of Arkansas, University of Michigan) review of the Singer-Blom procedures completed on 63 patients. In this series, five patients (8 per cent) were regarded as "voice failures" (p. 675). These patients were unable to produce "fluent tracheoesophageal speech despite adequate clinical trial" (p. 675). Finally, Donegan, Gluckman, and Singh (1981) report a one year experience with 23 patients. From a speech perspective, these authors classified the rehabilitation outcome as successful "if the patient attained fluent and intelligible speech" (p. 495). Donegan and colleagues indicated that "only three of our failures were due to inability to produce fluent speech" (p. 496).

The Singer-Blom method is a *speech* restoration technique. Hence, a criterion by which the outcome of this method must be evaluated is efficiency and proficiency of speech production. Published accounts of outcome using speech criteria certainly indicate that the Singer-Blom approach represents an important advance. It appears that many patients undergoing this form of treatment develop speech that is characterized as "fluent and intelligible." Moreover, a significant number of them develop speech quickly, and many of them were previously unable to produce fluent or intelligible discourse using esophageal speech produced on a conventional basis, which suggests a significant advance in treatment regimens available to laryngectomized patients.

The problems associated with evaluation of treatment outcomes are numerous and are not unique to this field of endeavor. One major problem associated with the interpretation of published reviews of speech outcomes of this method relates to the failure to carefully specify speech and vocal outcomes. Methodologies are available that permit valid, reliable specification of speech and vocal attributes and proficiency levels. It is regrettable, therefore, that more specific, replicable forms of speech assessment were not undertaken on the patient series reviewed to date.

A second problem relates to an apparent failure to clearly distinguish the differences between the terms *voice* and *speech*. The Singer-Blom technique or similar techniques (e.g., Panje, 1981) represent *speech* restoration approaches. Virtually all the titles of papers dealing with these approaches (see References) identify the voice restoration aspects of the procedure. Although human voice production represents an essential part of the speech act, this multidimensional part of speech production is but one piece of an even larger, multidimensional communication process. Hence, future specification of outcomes for these methods might well define outcomes in terms of both vocal and speech communication efficiency, attributes, and proficiency.

In this context, there is the related issue of ascertaining and distinguishing influences of surgical-prosthetic intervention from those occasioned by associated behavioral or nonsurgical influences. To put it simply, the ultimate success or level of proficiency achieved by patients undergoing puncture-type methods of treatment is not solely dependent upon the surgical procedure or upon surgical-prosthetic interactions. Rather, outcomes are dictated by complex interactions among surgical, prosthetic, behavioral, and nonmedical therapeutic influences. The interactions among these influences merit more careful study and appreciation.

Finally, there is the important investigative advantage afforded by the development of puncture-type methods. These methods offer minimally invasive entry for monitoring key respiratory influences on speech and vocal production. The advent of puncture-type methods opens the door for the completion of important investigations aimed at enriching the current understanding of mechanisms underlying the regulation of essential aspects of alaryngeal voice (e.g., vocal fundamental frequency and intensity) and speech (e.g., prosody) production.

NONSPEECH OUTCOMES

The tracheal puncture approach necessitates the creation of a connection between the trachea and the esophagus, the placement of a one-way valve into this connection, and the use of this surgical-prosthetic, pulmonary-digestive link to energize esophageal speech production. Successful culmination and continued use of this process of producing alaryngeal speech depends upon factors other than speech and voice limitation or failure.

Donegan and colleagues (1981) have addressed this issue succinctly. They state:

> A successful outcome was considered achieved if the patient attained fluent and intelligible speech *and* was willing and able to maintain the prosthesis unaided. Inability to achieve these goals was regarded as a failure. . . . We have included willingness and ability to maintain the prosthesis in the criteria for success. We feel this is necessary in that reporting results as fluency of speech only is not a true indication of how well these patients achieve vocal rehabilitation. Of the 23 patients in this series, 13 were deemed successful (56%), and there were 10 failures. Seven of the failures were due to the patients' inability to care for the prosthesis in a home setting despite having achieved fluent speech. The problems encountered included difficulty manipulating the prosthesis into position after cleaning and difficulty maintaining the prosthesis in position, and a few simply left the prosthesis out for prolonged periods allowing the fistula to close (pp. 495–496).

Donegan and colleagues (1981) acknowledge that the Singer-Blom technique "represents a dramatic advance in neoglottic surgery" (pp.

495–496), but they identified several nonspeech factors that may limit success or contribute to failure. In their series of 23 patients, 13 (56 per cent) were classified successful, whereas 10 were regarded as failures. Among the failure group, 7 failed because of factors unrelated to speech or vocal failure.

These patients were unable to care for the prosthesis despite having "fluent speech." Similar observations have been made by others. For example, Wetmore, Johns, and Baker (1981) noted that although 56 (89 per cent) of the 63 patients in their series developed speech, only 45 (71 per cent) have continued to use this modality. The main reasons for discontinuing use of this speech technique were inadvertent dislodgement of the prosthesis with subsequent closure of the TEP tract or patient noncompliance. Two patients in this series failed to use tracheoesophageal speech because of problems with aspiration. Wetmore, Johns, and Baker noted that "a minor degree of aspiration developed in five additional patients; thus aspiration was treated by cauterizing the TEP tract" (p. 674).

Wood and colleagues (1981) also commented about nonspeech factors that may limit the outcome of the tracheoesophageal puncture technique. In this series from the Cleveland Clinic, two patients required repeat puncture for complete stenosis of the TEP tract following displacement of the prosthesis due to incorrect taping. One patient developed cervical cellulitis when the TEP was mistakenly placed too high in the trachea. One patient developed acute, symptomatic aspiration. This was resolved by use of "aggressive silver nitrate (AGNO3) cautery of the fistula tract and reduction in the size of the stent" (p. 494).

Finally, there is the Singer, Blom, and Haymaker (1981) series of 129 patients. In this group, nine patients were unable to maintain the voice prosthesis in spite of speech acquisition. Singer and colleagues commented thus:

> Routine maintenance involves daily stoma hygiene, cleaning the prosthesis, and replacement with prescribed skin adhesives. Patients previously unable or unwilling to care for their tracheostomas were limited in their ability to handle the voice prosthesis. Visual problems, generalized infirmity, or disinterest precluded satisfactory adaptation to this method of vocal rehabilitation. Three patients with exceptionally low tracheostomas failed to use the prosthesis over time. In this group of failures, the prosthesis was removed and the puncture spontaneously closed in 12 to 24 hours. (p. 498)

These authors also commented

> Approximately 20% of the patients will experience occasional extrusion of the voice prosthesis, requiring replacement after dilatation of the tracheoesophageal puncture, and additional supervision of their stoma care regimen. Two of the patients accidently aspirated the voice prosthesis without consequence. The prostheses were retrieved with a flexible fiberoptic bronchoscope.

Problems relating to the tracheoesophageal puncture procedure have remained minimal. One patient developed cervical subcutaneous emphysema after he inadvertently removed the stent. There have been four marked inflammatory reactions around the stoma in irradiated patients. This problem required the use of a silicone tracheal vent tube or laryngectomy tube until the reaction resolved.

The most important group of problems is related to tracheal reflux. Although salivary contamination of the trachea can be a serious problem, no patients experienced aspiration pneumonia. Two patients had intractable leakage around the voice prosthesis and required a second procedure to close the puncture. Intermittent aspiration was reported by three patients three months to one year postoperatively. They were treated by repeated applications of electrocautery to the tracheoesophageal puncture to enhance stenosis. Nine others experienced minimal leakage which has been eliminated by a single application of electrocautery. (p. 498)

As indicated earlier, the problems associated with evaluation of the outcomes of surgical-prosthetic techniques are numerous and are not unique to this field of endeavor. It is apparent that, at a minimum, outcome must be evaluated in terms of both speech and nonspeech criteria. In recognition of this reality, Wood and colleagues (1981) offer patient criteria that they believe "largely determine the success or failure of this particular surgical procedure" (p. 492). Their criteria include adequate motivation and reasonable patient expectations; capacity of patients to learn; adequate manual dexterity and vision; adequate stomal size, maturity, and architecture; adequate physical health; and positive air insufflation test results.

Identification of these criteria highlights the fact that all patient series reviewed here embody sampling bias. Namely, patients considered for tracheoesophageal puncture are evaluated and are selected (or rejected) to undergo surgery and prosthetic management on some bases. This bias may exert a significant influence upon the outcome and makes comparative evaluation difficult to achieve.

Panje (1981) has addressed this problem. He indicated that "patient selection can significantly bias the end results to the point of misleading the observer to the effectiveness of the treatment or technique. Just as the attainment of esophageal speech is markedly influenced by patient anatomy, interest, intelligence and habits, so might these factors influence the success of prosthetic vocal rehabilitation" (pp. 118–119).

It is apparent that the tracheoesophageal puncture approach to speech restoration for laryngectomized patients represents a dramatic advance. Although this is true, the method is characterized by some relative liabilities. Thus, as is the case for esophageal speech and speech powered by artificial larynges, surgical-prosthetic assisted forms of speech are also not characterized by functional universality.

ESOPHAGEAL AIR INSUFFLATION TESTING

As part of the preoperative evaluation protocol used to assess a patient's candidacy for tracheoesophageal puncture, Singer and Blom (1980) have advocated routine, preoperative esophageal air insufflation testing. They stated

> The voice failures can be predicted preoperatively by the air insufflation test. The test is critical to successful patient selection. Limitation to airflow by this test correlated well with lack of initial voice fluency and the need for reeducation of the pharyngoesophageal muscles for voice production. To date there have been both false positives and negatives, but in limited numbers. We use the test as a relative guide to patient selection, and estimation of time involved for postsurgical rehabilitation. (p. 532)

Blom, Singer, and Haymaker (1982) commented that "in spite of a patent tracheoesophageal puncture and functional voice prosthesis, 16 patients failed to develop satisfactory speech. All were assessed by preoperative insufflation of the esophagus with voice failure correlating with complete cessation of airflow during speech or brisk esophageal distention. The 16 patients were predicted by insufflation" (p. 576). Thirteen additional patients exhibited limitation to airflow or lack of fluency, but they eventually acquired satisfactory tracheoesophageal speech.

These observations raise questions about the validity of the assertion that "voice failures can be predicted preoperatively by the air insufflation test (Singer and Blom, 1980)" (p. 552). Indeed, Donegan and colleagues (1981) have written that all patients in their series "were assessed preoperatively by the surgeon and the speech therapist. The air insufflation test was used in all patients in an attempt to predict the outcome of the procedure, but was found to be of limited value in predicting success or failure of the tracheoesophageal puncture" (p. 495).

Wood and colleagues (1981) relate that they "continue to use the air insufflation test for prognostic purposes despite a number of false-positive results" (p. 492). Panje (1981) has commented that "the air insufflation test has been advocated by some as a determinant of those patients who will do best with tracheoesophageal sound production. . . . However, both patients who failed to develop speech with Voice Button placement had had sound production on the administration of air into the esophagus via a small catheter, which seems to demonstrate the capricious nature of the test and the variability among patients" (p. 119).

It is clear that all "failures" may not be predicted preoperatively by air insufflation testing, although this form of testing does identify a subgroup of patients who cannot achieve airflow across the pharyngoesophagus during catheter-induced air insufflation and esophageal distention. Important questions are raised by the advocacy of esophageal air insufflation testing and the notation of variable responses to this form of assessment of pharyngoesophageal function. For example, what is the rate of prediction offered by preoperative air insufflation testing? Precisely what is predicted (e.g., ability to produce voice, sustain voice, use voice appropriately as part of the speech act)? In addition, specific details are needed on just how the air insufflation tests are conducted since there is a need to determine whether procedural variables used in the administration of this test influence outcome of test results.

SELECTIVE MYOTOMY FOR VOICE RESTORATION

Speech and surgical specialists have often expressed the view that improvement in the rate and efficiency of voice reacquisition with esophageal phonation might occur if consideration was given to surgically altering the anatomy and physiology of the pharyngoesophageal (PE) segment. Singer and Blom (1981) have raised some provocative issues about the consequences of surgical alteration of the PE segment by proposing selective myotomy for voice restoration after total laryngectomy.

The observations of Singer and Blom (1981) have shown that some laryngectomized patients cannot achieve airflow across the pharyngoesophagus in association with insufflation of air into the esophagus, that parapharyngeal nerve block enabled these patients to temporarily achieve airflow across the pharyngoesophagus, and that selective, unilateral myotomy of the pharyngeal constrictors enabled these patients to achieve airflow across the pharyngoesophagus, produce voice, and achieve speech fluency. These observations emphasize the role played by altered function of the PE segment in influencing reacquisition of voice and speech following total laryngectomy, and they highlight the potential contribution surgical alteration of the PE segment may make to the voice and speech reacquisition process.

The observations made by Singer and Blom (1981) also raise some provocative questions. For example, they concluded that "airflow induced spasm of the cricopharyngeus and pharyngeal constrictor muscles seems to be an important factor in failures of more patients to acquire fluent speech" (p. 673). There appears to be little question about the fact that insufflation of air into the esophagus, coupled with esophageal distention, is associated with PE segment closure that is air tight in some laryngectomized patients. Although this is true, important issues related to this fact remain unclear.

For example, it is not known whether this form of air tight closure is induced by air flow. If flow cannot be passed across the pharyngoesophagus, such an explanation is doubtful. Other questions include determining the mechanisms underlying the production of air tight closure of the upper esophageal sphincter. Precisely how can or does the "air-filled and distended esophagus stimulate cricopharyngeal and pharyngeal constrictor muscle contraction?" (Singer and Blom, 1980 p. 673). How is this air tight response mediated? Is this response related to the method of surgical closure? Further consideration of the response of the normal PE sphincter to esophageal distention and air insufflation testing of this type is needed. Should this air tight response properly be regarded as spasm? If so, what triggers this spasmodic behavior? There are additional questions about whether this response is abnormal and why only a relatively small percentage of sampled laryngectomized patients exhibit this response. What is special about this group or subsample? Finally, there is a need to clarify the rationale for routinely performing selective, unilateral myotomy when only some patients exhibit this "problem" and when the mechanism underlying this response remains unclear.

PROSTHESIS DESIGN AND FUNCTION

Puncture-type methods of speech restoration require the use of a one-way, tracheoesophageal puncture prosthesis. This prosthesis serves three primary functions: it maintains patency within the TEP; it permits air shunting between the trachea and the esophagus, and it functions as a one-way valve to prevent reflux of esophageal contents into the airway.

From a design perspective, tracheoesophageal puncture prostheses should be minimally resistive to airflow through them from the trachea to the esophagus, and maximally resistive to the flow of material entering the device from the esophagus. Minimal airway resistance of these prostheses to air flowing through them would be expected to enhance the efficiency of esophageal voice and speech production, while maximal resistance to flow reversal would attest to the competency of the device as a one-way valve.

At the time of this writing, two one-way valved prostheses have been developed for use in puncture-type approaches to speech rehabilitation. Singer and Blom (1980) have developed a duckbill prosthesis, while Panje (1981) has developed a four-flutter or flap, valved prosthesis. Both of these devices have apparently been developed on an empirical basis.

The opposition Singer-Blom prostheses offer to the flow of air through them has been calculated (Moon, Sullivan, and Weinberg, 1983; Weinberg, Horii, Blom, and Singer, 1982). The results of these works reveal that the overall airway resistance Singer-Blom prostheses offer to air flow is about 125 cm H_2O/LPS and that the overall resistance of these prostheses remains relatively constant as a function of increasing flow rate (0.05 to 0.2 LPS range). Average airway resistance for Singer-Blom prostheses is in excess of three times that offered by the normal human larynx during vowel production.

Weinberg (1982) has recently also calculated the resistance offered by prostheses developed by Panje (1981). The results of this work revealed that the opposition of Panje devices to airflow through them is more substantial. Resistance values for individual Voice Button prostheses ranged from 285 to 440 cm H_2O/LPS. These resistance values are higher than those calculated for opposition offered by esophageal voicing sources, suggesting that patients using Panje Voice Buttons may have to work more to overcome prosthetic opposition of air flow than they would to excite and sustain vibration of their voicing source. This situation would be expected to result in impoverished and inefficient production of voice and speech and it highlights the potential for modification in prosthesis design (Weinberg, 1982).

Further analysis of prosthesis function is expected to provide fundamental data critical to enlarging understanding of voice and speech production used by patients who speak with puncture methods, and to provide information essential to the future development of prosthesis modification. Tracheoesophageal puncture prostheses have apparently been developed on an empirical basis. Thus, basic studies aimed at defining the essential attributes of valve function are needed. These attributes can be studied using modeling approaches and computer-assisted design methods. It is expected that the results of such basic work will lead to enlightened understanding of prosthesis function and suggest potential modifications likely to enhance vocal and speech efficiency or valve competency. Basic studies of valve competency to combat flow reversal have apparently not yet been conducted.

As part of the general approach to developing a puncture-type method of speech restoration, Blom, Singer, and Haymaker (1982) have also developed a lightweight, two-way respiratory valve. This device permits two-way airflow at the stoma for vegetative breathing and converts to a one-way inspiratory valve with increased airflow. In the latter circumstance, air is diverted into the esophagus, eliminating the need for finger occlusion of the stoma. This device would be expected to represent a significant advance. The development of this device has also proceeded on an empirical basis, and basic research is needed before firm conclusions regarding its usefulness, function, or redesign can be made.

SPEECH PATHOLOGY: ROLES AND CONTRIBUTIONS

The recent development of tracheoesophageal puncture-type approaches to speech restoration in no way diminishes the role of speech pathologists in the rehabilitation process offered to laryngectomized patients. Although these advances alter some of the functions speech pathologists play in this process, the contributions made by speech pathologists to rehabilitation continue to play a critical role.

As indicated earlier, puncture-type approaches to restoration represent speech reacquisition methods. The ultimate success of these methods depends primarily upon interactions, yet unspecified, among surgical, prosthetic, behavioral, and nonmedical therapeutic factors. The process of speech rehabilitation for patients using puncture-type methods involves far more than merely "restoring the voice or getting the voice back."

This writer is concerned about the apparently limited therapeutic management offered to patients undergoing tracheoesophageal puncture-type, surgical-prosthetic forms of treatment. The published reports reviewed in earlier sections of this chapter deal solely with the role of speech pathologists in patient selection, prosthesis fitting, and *voice* restoration. There is ample evidence to support this writer's view that the process of speech production is profoundly altered in patients who undergo these procedures. Restoration of speech involves much more than merely getting the voice back. Hence, speech pathologists must, at a minimum, routinely manage rate and temporal characteristics, enhance articulation and intelligibility attributes, eliminate extraneous behaviors and noises, and perfect realization of prosody and linguistic contrasts in patients who have undergone surgical-prosthetic treatment (see Weinberg, 1983, for details).

Speech pathologists who fail to address these facets of speech communication management may fail to fully comprehend speech restoration for laryngectomized patients and may seriously underestimate the contributions therapy can provide. This writer firmly believes that speech management dealing merely with prosthesis fitting and early voice return seriously undercuts the ultimate levels of speech proficiency that patients undergoing forms of surgical-prosthetic treatment might reasonably be expected to achieve. A comprehensive program of therapy must be offered and delivered to such patients (see Weinberg, 1983, for details). This program need not be long, however.

Clearly, therapy devoted solely to prosthesis fitting and voice return will lead to serious undercutting. On the other hand, efficient therapy devoted to patient selection, prosthesis fitting, voice return, *and* aspects of speech communication common to other forms of normal and alaryngeal speech would be expected to increase the prevalence of highly proficient alaryngeal speakers at the conclusion of speech rehabilitation. Further, speech pathologists can also contribute substantially to the improved development of sensitive and reliable outcome measures, so lacking in current reports. Failure to address speech rehabilitation in a comprehensive form seems likely to result in compromise and in diminished ultimate levels of speech attainment.

CONCLUSION

In this offering, some contemporary advances in the field of speech rehabilitation for laryngectomized patients have been reviewed. The more significant advances in this field are those related to surgical-prosthetic management. In addition to identifying advances in this field of endeavor, several important issues and questions raised by these advances have also been identified. It is clear that the field of speech rehabilitation for laryngectomized patients continues to be an exciting one. Advances have been made in both basic understanding and clinical application. It is hoped that in addition to providing information, the material discussed here will serve to interest others in the diverse problems associated with speech restoration following total laryngectomy, stimulate additional participation in this exciting arena of basic and applied research and rehabilitation, and highlight the need for continued interdisciplinary cooperation so essential to the improved quality of future rehabilitation of laryngectomized patients.

REFERENCES

Blom, E. D., Singer, M. I., and Haymaker, R. C. (1982). Tracheostoma valve for postlaryngectomy voice rehabilitation. *Annals of Otology, Rhinology, and Laryngology, 91,* 576–578.

Donegan, J. O., Gluckman, J. L., and Singh, J. (1981). Limitations of the Blom-Singer technique for voice restoration. *Annals of Otology, Rhinology, and Laryngology, 90,* 495–497.

Gandour, J., and Weinberg, B. (1983). Perception of intonational contrasts in alaryngeal speech. *Journal of Speech and Hearing Research, 26,* 142–148.

Gandour, J., and Weinberg, B. (1982). Perception of contrastive stress in alaryngeal speech. *Journal of Phonetics, 10,* 347–350.

Gandour, J., Weinberg, B., and Garzione, B. (1983). Perception of lexical stresss in alaryngeal speech. *Journal of Speech and Hearing Research, 26,* 418–424.

Gandour, J., Weinberg, B., and Kosowsky, A. (1983). Perception of syntactic stress in alaryngeal speech. *Language and Speech, 25,* 299–304.

McHenry, M., Reich, A., and Minifie, F. (1982). Acoustical characteristics of intended syllabic stress in excellent esophageal speakers. *Journal of Speech and Hearing Research, 25,* 564–753.

Moon, J.B., Sullivan, J., and Weinberg, B. (1983). Evaluations of Blom-Singer tracheoesophageal puncture prostheses. *Journal of Speech and Hearing Research, 26,* 459–464.

Panje, W. R. (1981). Prosthetic vocal rehabilitation following laryngectomy. *Annals of Otology, Rhinology, and Laryngology, 90,* 116–120.

Scarpino, J., and Weinberg, B. (1981). Junctural contrasts in esophageal and normal speech. *Journal of Speech and Hearing Research, 46,* 120–126.

Shedd, D. P., and Weinberg, B. (1980). *Surgical-prosthetic approaches to speech rehabilitation.* Boston: G. K. Hall.

Singer, M. I., and Blom, E. D. (1980). An endoscopic technique for restoration of voice after laryngectomy. *Annals of Otology, Rhinology and Laryngology, 89,* 529–533.

Singer, M. I., and Blom, E. D. (1981). Selective myotomy for voice restoration after total laryngectomy. *Archives of Otolaryngology, 107,* 670–673.

Singer, M. I., Blom, E. D., and Haymaker, R. C. (1981). Further experience with voice restoration after total laryngectomy. *Annals of Otology, Rhinology, and Laryngology, 90,* 498–502.

Weinberg, B. (1980). *Readings in speech following total laryngectomy.* Baltimore: University Park Press.

Weinberg, B. (1982). Airway resistance of the Voice Button. *Archives of Otolaryngology, 108,* 498–500.

Weinberg, B. (1983). Speech and voice restoration following total laryngectomy. In W. H. Perkins (Ed.), *Current Therapy in Communication Disorders* (Vol. 4). New York: Thieme-Stratton.

Weinberg, B., Horii, Y., Blom, E., and Singer, M. (1982). Airway resistance during esophageal phonation. *Journal of Speech and Hearing Disorders, 47,* 194–199.

Wetmore, S. J., Johns, M. E., and Baker, S. H. (1981). The Singer-Blom voice restoration procedure. *Archives of Otolaryngology, 107,* 674–676.

Wood, B. G., Rusnov, M. G., Tucker, H. M., and Levine, H. L. (1981). Tracheoesophageal puncture for alaryngeal voice restoration. *Annals of Otology, Rhinology, and Laryngology, 90,* 492–494.

Chapter 6

Voice Disorders: The Measurement of Clinical Progress

Thomas S. Johnson

Evaluation and treatment of voice disorders has had a long and curious development, with its roots primarily in vocal music and with some input from early medical science. Its strong connection with the musical and theatrical arts has greatly affected the contemporary practices of voice therapy (Brodnitz, 1971; Moore, 1977). Concurrent, sometimes controversial philosophies grew from those advocating a more symptomatic approach to vocal behavior and those who held that voice disturbance was reflective of personality disturbance. Hence, a wide variety of therapy approaches emerged, some of which have seemed foreign and strange to practicing speech-language pathologists. Symptomatic treatments were generally adapted from general speech, vocal music and theater, while psychiatric medicine contributed the personality theories. The belief held by a number of early writers that the voice is the "mirror of the emotions" and that it plays an important role in revealing information about the fears, anxieties, and emotional struggles of the individual (Brodnitz, 1971; Moses, 1954) has contributed significantly to the development of current evaluative and therapeutic processes for the management of voice problems.

Moore (1977), in his excellent and thought-provoking treatise on the major issues in voice disorders, reviewed 50 years of research and practice and made comparisons between then contemporary textbook writings in voice disorders and several classic publications of earlier years. His discussion indicated the following:

> Four features stand out in the recent publications: (1) voice disorders are described in greater detail and reflect an increased understanding of basic problems, but the problems are the same; (2) more attention is paid to specific vocal disorders such as laryngectomy; (3) there is a greater variety of therapeutic techniques; and (4) the major emphases in therapy remain as before: training in breath control (where indicated), relaxation and reduction of laryngeal

tension, training in listening, articulatory adjustments, and special techniques. These are applied to deviations in pitch, intensity, and quality (including the resonance disorders). Obviously, not much change in the basic clinical practices appears to have occurred over the years. (p. 156)

It is striking that the same conclusion could be drawn five years later from a review of more recent titles in the field. In completing such a review, the following conclusions were drawn: greater detail is available; still more attention is given special problems (especially spastic dysphonia); a somewhat increased variety of therapeutic techniques (though not greatly different) are described; and the major emphases remain essentially the same with the addition of some behavioral approaches and programmed formats. Current evaluation and therapeutic practices have been comprehensively described in recent years by Aronson (1980), Boone (1977), Cooper and Cooper (1977), Filter (1982b), Greene (1980), Murry (1982), and Wilson (1979). Contemporary voice therapy packaged kits have also been developed by Wilson and Rice (1977), Polow and Kaplan (1979), and Boone (1981). No attempt in this chapter will be made to review fundamental therapy approaches, as they are already available in these publications, and it is not the author's desire to add to the glut of restated, redescribed, widely known therapeutics.

The big disappointment with all of these publications is a significant lack of research data applied to validate the described clinical methodologies. Research on the clinical effectiveness of voice therapy procedures is regrettably sparse (Johnson, 1974; Michel and Wendahl, 1971; Moore, 1977; Reed, 1980). The overwhelming number of evaluative and treatment procedures described by the authors named have not been subjected to rigorous clinical research and contain few reports of precise data substantiating their effectiveness.

In recent years the field of communication disorders has experienced a demand for increased accountability. Such clinical accountability requires the development and use of objective measurement procedures (Reed, 1980). In the area of voice disorders, there has been a lack of such measurement techniques, and hence the therapeutic management of voice problems has had few accountability data available to it (Johnson, 1974; Lubker, 1979; Michel and Wendahl, 1971; Reed, 1980). Voice evaluation and measurement have long been practical problems for the voice clinician. Hence, the evaluative capability of clinicians has been limited chiefly to descriptive procedures, using subjective adjectives or adverbs, which have attempted to describe the acoustic perceptions of the voice. Such terms as hoarse, harsh, rough, sandy, breathy, and metallic, as well as many others (Laver, 1968; Perkins, 1971), have been used to describe the acoustic product of pathologic laryngeal physiology. Other descriptive systems have been proposed, but they suffer a lack of intra- and interexaminer reliability and are not sensitive to progressive change during voice management. Wilson's (1972) system offers descriptive information that is helpful in relating in a general way to the physiology of the laryngeal structures; however, agreement between judges is, in the author's experience, difficult to obtain, even using Wilson's prescribed training (Wilson and Rice, 1977). Additionally, other physiologic measures have simply not been precise enough or sensitive enough to the changes desired and those of most interest to the voice clinician. Further, a lack of standardization of evaluation procedures and a concurrent scarcity of normative data on vocal parameters also contribute to the imprecision of currently applied procedures to voice evaluation and measurement. An additional contributing force to this measurement dilemma faced by the voice clinician has been the historical reliance by the clinician on medical evaluation, chiefly that of indirect laryngoscopy. Even from a medical perspective, indirect laryngoscopy is at best an imprecise procedure, particularly for the purpose of reporting progress or improvement towards remediation of a laryngeal problem. The fleeting moment of visual observation interpreted through the subjective perception of the medical practitioner is not a very satisfactory procedure for monitoring laryngeal change over time. Recent advances in flexible fiberoptic systems hold promise in this regard; however, at present this technology is available only in larger medical facilities. The voice clinician then must look elsewhere to find a more satisfactory technique for achieving clinical accountability in voice therapy. The most exciting recent advances in the area of voice disorders, in the author's view, are investigations of the parameters of vocal functioning and of establishing ways and means of measuring them. For the first time, the profession is at the threshold of being able to validate years of clinical practice in voice disorders with efficient data collection techniques. These recent advances are the focus of the chapter to follow.

VOICE AS BEHAVIOR

The aforementioned notion that the voice is somehow the "mirror of the emotions" or the "barometer of the soul" seems to have created an aura about the voice that implies it is somehow different or in some ways mysterious and hence requires the use of mysterious procedures to correct it. One of the most important recent advances in the management of voice problems is the consideration that voice is behavior and is subject to what we know about the modification of, and change in, other types of behavior. In short, voice behaviors are classes of behaviors, which can be shaped and modified by use of principles of applied behavior analysis (Costello, 1977; Johnson, 1974; Miller, 1980; Mowrer, 1982).

In recent years, applied behavior analysis technology seems to have profoundly affected in all areas of educational intervention, including communicative disorders (Mowrer, 1982; Perkins, 1971). This movement has also had an impact on the management of voice disorders. Nell (1968) was the first writer who viewed the potential applicability of this evolving technology to voice problems. Hunsaker (1970) reported data on its applicability with a single subject, and other authors subsequently reported data indicating that vocal behaviors and behaviors associated with voice were manipulable response classes (Beck, 1976; Beste, 1971; Drudge and Phillips, 1976; Johnson, 1985; Parrish, 1972; Pierce, 1974; Rothwell, 1974; Smee, 1974). This finding allowed a rationale to develop, bringing the measurement of specific vocal behaviors into the context of "vocal hyperfunction" as originally proposed by Froeschels (1952) and augmented by Brodnitz (1971). In short, if vocal hyperfunction (i.e., vocal misuse and abuse) is responsible for a large majority of voice problems, as is argued by Brodnitz (1971), Perkins (1971), Boone (1977), Greene (1980), and others, then these abusive behaviors should be able to be accurately pinpointed, recorded, and subjected to experimental manipulation such as that advocated in the applied behavior analysis strategy.

MODIFICATION OF HYPERFUNCTIONAL VOCAL BEHAVIOR

Most vocal problems in both children and adults have been primarily related to use, misuse, and abuse of the vocal mechanisms (hyperfunctional behaviors). The concept of vocal hyperfunction includes any behaviors that result in excessive muscular tension in the vocal tract. This excessive tension may come from any of the variety of vocal behaviors that induce tension into the vocal tract at any level. The laryngeal mechanism is largely a muscular system and functions in the same way as other muscular systems in the body in relation to hyperfunctional usage. To use the analogy of running and the muscular system of the legs, an individual could abuse or misuse the leg muscles in several ways: by running normally too long, or running too hard, or running in an abnormal fashion, putting too much stress on one leg or the other. Each of these activities could lead to a hyperfunctioning leg muscle system. The analogy holds true also for use of the vocal musculature. Additionally, prolonged hyperfunctioning of a muscle system fatigues the muscles to the degree that they finally become unable to produce a normal degree of muscle tone, and the condition of hypofunction sets in. As hypofunction increases, the muscular effort must also increase, adding more hyperfunctional usage to the system and fatiguing the muscles even more as the condition increases in severity in a vicious spiral. In laryngeal functioning, prolonged hyperfunctional use of the voice fatigues the vocal musculature to the degree that the muscles are unable to produce a normal degree of muscle tone, and a degree of hypofunction sets in. This hypofunction causes the vocal musculature to work even harder at producing appropriate phonation and in doing so adds more hyperfunction behavior, thus further fatiguing the musculature. More effort is added, and the condition worsens. This combined process of hyper- and hypofunctioning is an interesting phenomenon in the larynx, especially because the hyperfunctional behavior can also lead to the formation of organic-structural changes (such as nodules, thickened cords, and polyps) on the margins of the vocal folds. This further complicates the process and consequently affects the level of effort required for vocal fold functioning because of the increased mass of the folds generated by the presence of these vocal pathologies.

Several additional factors may interplay in this process of hyperfunction to produce a "hyperfunctional voice problem." These factors are susceptibility factors and relate to predisposing characteristics of the person with hyperfunctional vocal behavior. The combination of these susceptibility factors with hyperfunctional behavior (i.e., use, abuse, misuse) of the laryngeal mechanism can result in the formation of laryngeal pathologies and in the presence of vocal symptoms. Susceptibility factors include histologic differences in the basic cellular makeup of the individual laryngeal mechanisms, the presence of an invading bacterial or viral organism, the physical conditioning history of the individual's laryngeal mechanism, and other such factors that could increase an individual's susceptibility to the development of laryngeal problems. Figure 6-1 presents hypothetical examples of the combination of susceptibility factors and hyperfunctional behaviors in a general hyperfunctional equation relationship.

In Example 1, the individual has not conditioned his or her voice properly and then overuses the voice in singing, resulting in laryngeal inflammation and vocal disturbance. This example is representative of frequently seen cases in which voice majors who come to college with little vocal training or experience throw themselves completely into vocal

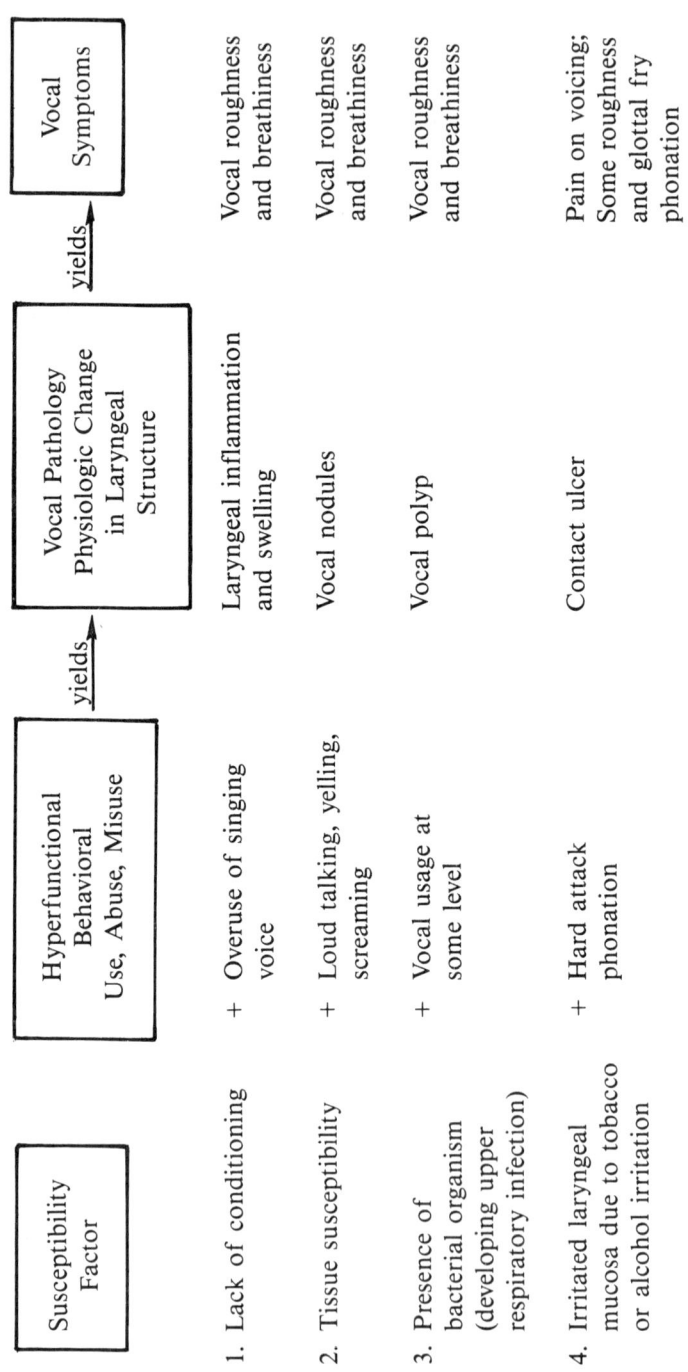

Figure 6-1. The hyperfunctional equation with four hypothetical examples of how it works.

performance and practice with little thought about the need to condition the vocal musculature. This situation is analogous to the nonrunner who decides to run in a marathon race with little though beforehand about a long and intensive program of physical conditioning.

Example 2 represents the frequently seen school child who seems not to yell or scream any more than his or her peers, but whose larynx has developed a set of vocal nodules. Histologic differences may be present in the individual larynx, and it is my (as yet unproved) hypothesis that such differences may ultimately account for one child developing nodules while another does not, when their levels of usage are strikingly similar.

Examples 3 and 4 provide additional hypothetical examples of how the hyperfunctional cycle can work to cause vocal problems.

The modification of hyperfunctional problems necessitates interrupting the hyperfunctional cycle and reducing the amount of potential hyperfunctional behavior, which, along with the susceptibility factors, has produced the vocal pathology. The clinician must remain aware and conscious of the susceptibility factors in planning and carrying out appropriate therapy procedures and, in some instances (e.g., lack of conditioning), build components into the total therapeutic plan to handle such factors.

The technology of applied behavior analysis suggests that behaviors be precisely defined so that they can be observed and counted readily. In attempting to interrupt the hyperfunctional cycle and reduce the amount of potential hyperfunctional behavior, the clinician needs to pinpoint carefully which of the client's behaviors is primarily responsible for the voice problem. Once the contributory behavior or behaviors are pinpointed precisely, and a baseline of those behaviors is obtained over a selected time, then the clinician must select a strategy to reduce the rate of occurrence of those behaviors. Respective pinpointed hyperfunction-producing behaviors associated with these problems include behaviors involved in phonation, respiration, and resonation. Specific examples include yelling, loud talking, coughing, throat clearing, strained phonation, hard attack phonation, pharyngeal tightness, inappropriate tongue carriage, restricted mouth opening, speaking on expiratory reserve air, and inadequate breath support.

In 1976, the author published a data-based program, the Vocal Abuse Reduction Program (VARP), based on seven years of supportive single-subject design research (Johnson, 1985). This program used a self-control management strategy from applied behavior analysis with a sensitive data collection procedure in the form of daily behavioral charting to produce a replicable, valid therapeutic procedure for affecting the reduction of hyperfunctional voice behaviors. The VARP also gave the clinician the opportunity to monitor progress continuously over the course of therapy by viewing the daily behavior records of vocally abusive behaviors. The VARP is a clinical management program that pinpoints vocal abuse and misuse behaviors for each client with such behaviors resulting in the formation of laryngeal pathologies (i.e., nodules, polyps, contact ulcers, and thickened cords), systematically and precisely reduces the pinpointed vocal abuse behaviors in specific high probability situations or time periods, and reduces or eliminates the abuse-generated laryngeal pathology and makes possible the establishment of normal voice quality. The VARP program is described in detail by Johnson (1984, 1985).

Figure 6–2 presents an example of the daily behavior chart obtained when the VARP program is used. The record indicates the rate of occurrence of abuse and misuse behaviors in selected time periods, which are gradually increased in length as control is obtained in each situation. The data themselves represent data collected by the client, who counts his or her own abuse and misuse behaviors with the assistance of a wrist counter.

This chart presents "yells" and "loud talk" behaviors occurring during specified situations over a 12 week management program with VARP. During the first 2 weeks, the behaviors were self monitored only during the morning recess period at school (20 minutes of monitored time). During weeks 3 and 4, the monitoring time was extended to include afternoon recess (totaling 35 minutes of monitored time). The magnitude of change during these first 4 weeks ranges from 1.7 behaviors per minute (or 34 yells–loud talks in 20 minutes) on the first data day to 0 yells–loud talk behaviors in 35 minutes on the final day of the fourth week. The rate of yelling and loud talking behavior may be seen to decelerate markedly during this period as a consequence of self-monitoring of those behaviors. In the fifth week, the monitored time is further extended to include a 35 minute lunch period (total monitored time, 70 minutes), with 3 days at the end of the week of no recorded yells or loud talk behaviors. In weeks 6 and 7, the time period is again extended to include after school until 6:00 PM, bringing the total monitored time to 220 minutes. Again, 3 days of no yells or loud talk behaviors appear at the end of week 7. The monitored time was then extended to include the entire day during weeks 8 through 12, with resulting low rates of yells and loud talk behaviors, including several full days of no self-observed loud talk and yell behaviors. On the third day of the eighth week, the client was seen by the laryngologist, who reported no remnant of the moderately large bilateral nodules. Rechecks by the examining laryngologist on the dates indicated at the top of the chart revealed no reoccurrence of the nodules. It is also interesting that good vocal quality did not return completely until the tenth week.

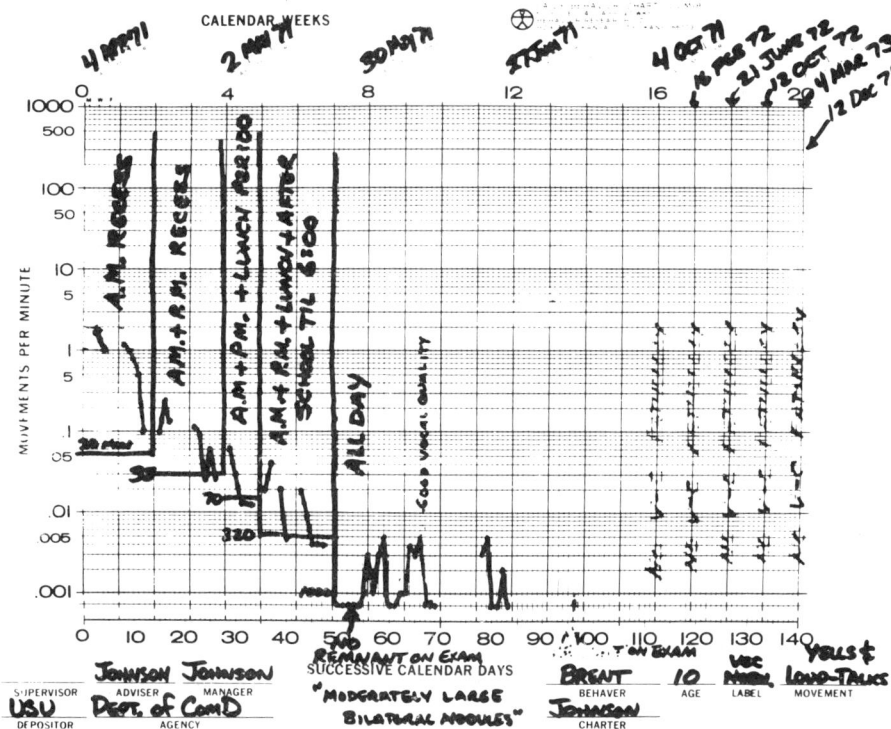

Figure 6-2. Example of daily behavioral chart of VARP intervention.

Intervention with VARP has been systematically studied in a series of similar single subject research projects at Utah State University. These successful systematic replications of VARP intervention have demonstrated the effectiveness and predictability of the VARP procedure.

Certainly, there are other methods for reducing hyperfunctional voice behaviors effectively; however, no reported procedures have the data base and predictive capability of the VARP procedure. For example, Wilson and Rice (1977) and Boone (1981) both describe abuse reduction programs but present no clinical data to support the procedures' effectiveness.

The recent interest in behavioral approaches to the study of the voice management process suggests some basic management principles.

1. Voice and voice disorders are not mysterious problems requiring unusual procedures to manage them effectively. Fundamental clinical processes are the same as those appropriate for communication disorders.

2. Voice and its associated features are behaviors. Hence, voice and the parameters relating to its physiology and pathology are not exempt from the principles of learning. Most voice problems spring from hyperfunctional action of the vocal mechanism, and these behaviors can be modified by applied behavior analysis procedures.

3. Some voice disorders have primarily an organic basis. Even so, the therapeutic and evaluative procedures used to facilitate a better voice can take advantage of what is known about the modification of behavior. This fact has been largely neglected in the voice therapy literature.

4. The utilization of careful stimulus programming, control, and precise consequence management is as facilitative in voice therapy as it is in other areas of speech-language pathology.

These principles suggest that there are many potential applications of applied behavior analysis technology to voice problems, whether hyperfunctional in nature or of an organic origin. At present, there is a great lack of material in the voice literature regarding these potential applications (Mowrer, 1982). In his review of instructional programs in the field, Mowrer laments the lack of such developed programs for the treatment of voice disorders. Additionally, Johnson (1974), Moore (1977), and Reed (1980) have all addressed the serious lack of research data addressing fundamental therapeutic management questions. The recent report by Drudge and Phillips (1976) is cited by both Mowrer (1982) and Reed (1980) as an example of the type of research that is seriously needed in voice therapeutics. Their 31 step program was designed to accomplish four major goals: elimination of vocal abuse, easy initiation of phonation, increased clear phonation time, and increased loudness without increase in laryngeal tension. Their program was criterion referenced, and they presented data on three subjects who successfully completed the program. Other behavioral programmed approaches to the management of voice problems have been studied by Smee (1974), Coachbuilder (1972), Greiner (1973), and Vance (1976). Briefly, these studies used the extended length and complexity of utterance therapy strategy (Ryan, 1974) to program for pitch disorders and quality problems. Data presented in these studies indicated the effectiveness of the programmed approach to the problems studied.

CLINICAL ASSESSMENT OF LARYNGEAL FUNCTIONING

Reed (1980) indicated that the most fundamental need for voice research was to replace vague terms with measurable observations sensitive enough to allow the results to be interpreted by other investigators. Johnson (1974) echoed that concern and proposed a strategy and philosophy for what was termed a "functional voice evaluation format." Recently, Filter (1982b) reviewed much of the work completed in the voice evaluation area over the past several years. He described current case history procedures, screening procedures, perceptual description formats, associated behaviors, and additional data. Michel and Wendahl's (1971) landmark discussion concerning correlates of voice production suggested 12 parameters to be considered for investigation in the determination of pertinent measurable voice parameters. These 12 correlates form a basic set of measurable features of the voice, which, when investigated fully, could constitute a measurement battery to assess the adequacy of laryngeal or vocal functioning. Michel and Wendahl proposed "to present voice as a multidimensional series of measurable events, implying that a single phonation can be assessed in many different ways" (p. 267). The 12 correlates they proposed were vital capacity of the lungs, maximum duration of controlled sustained blowing, modal frequency level, maximum frequency ranges, maximum duration of sustained phonation, volume-velocity flow during phonation, glottal waveform, sound pressure level, jitter of the vocal signal, shimmer of the vocal signal, effort level (vocal), and transfer function of the vocal tract. Reed (1980), in discussing Michel and Wendahl's correlates, suggested six parameters that could serve as initial efforts to address the major concepts of voice quality: volume-velocity airflow, jitter, shimmer, effort level, electomyographic studies, and rise-fall time.

Since the 1960s, data from voice science laboratories have emerged signaling interest in the development of objective measurement parameters of the voice. An exhaustive review of this work is outside the scope of this chapter; however, much excellent laboratory work has yielded important information regarding the measurement of laryngeal function. Central to this work is that of Koike and colleagues (Hirano, Koike, and von Leden, 1968; Koike, 1968; Koike and Hirano, 1968; Koike, Hirano, and von Leden, 1967) Isshiki and associates (Isshiki, 1964, 1965; Isshiki, Okamura, and Morimoto, 1967; Isshiki, Okamura, Tanabe, and Morimoto, 1969; Isshiki and von Leden, 1964; Isshiki, Yanagihara, and Morimoto, 1966), Iwata and von Leden (1970), and Yanagihara and associates (Yanagihara and Koike, 1967; Yanagihara, Koike, and von Leden, 1966; Yanagihara and von Leden, 1967).

In another landmark article, Beckett (1971) suggested that several specific measures derived from the voice science laboratory could be clinically applied to patients with respirometric or voice disturbances. Additionally, he indicated that the respirometer was an effective, reliable means of obtaining those data clinically without the extensive instrumentation utilized in the voice science laboratory. Beckett proposed seven aerodynamic measures that could have diagnostic or clinical value. They included one-stage vital capacity (VC), phonation volume (PV), phonation time (PT), maximum predicted phonation time (MPT), mean flow rate (MFR), vocal velocity index (VVI), and phonation time–maximum predicted phonation time (PT/MPT).

Johnson and associates began in 1970 to apply such data gathering techniques on an experimental basis to clinical populations of voice disordered individuals, as well as to subjects without voice disorders. Initially, they conducted a series of studies that made use of precision measurement in combination with behavior modification techniques in persons with voice disorders (Beck, 1976; Hunsaker, 1970; Parrish, 1972; Pierce, 1974; Rothwell, 1974; Vance, 1976). These investigations culminated with the publishing of the Vocal Abuse Reduction Program as an effective data-based clinical voice management program (see earlier discussion). The cited thesis studies were single-subject design investigations of the effectiveness of the Vocal Abuse Reduction Program. With the establishment of this program as an effective, replicable, predictable clinical procedure, it became possible to utilize several experimental measurement procedures, as suggested by the work of Michel and Wendahl (1971) and that of Beckett (1971), for monitoring data as voice therapy progressed during VARP. Two investigators, Thompson (1976) and Smee (1974), demonstrated the feasibility of using experimental measurement procedures for monitoring client progress during voice management. This was done by tracking the measures over the course of treatment with several individual subjects, VARP being used as the intervention procedure.

Although the feasibility for the therapeutic tracking use of the procedure was demonstrated, the amount of information known about unimpaired performance on the individual measurements was minimal, and guideposts for interpreting the meaning of changes in those measurements were limited. Hence, a series of subsequent investigations was begun to study the use of these measures on the performance of varying age groups of children and adults without voice disorders (Child, 1979; Inglis, 1977; Lee, 1978; Taylor, 1980; Williams, 1977; Williams, 1979). The results of these investigations of subjects without voice disorders were summarized by Hammond (1981). The measurements included in the battery selected for study were vital capacity (VC), phonation volume (PV), phonation time (PT), phonation time ratio (PTR), maximum flow rate (MFR), phonation quotient (PQ), vocal velocity index (VVI), and phonation volume–vital capacity ratio (PV/VC). As indicated previously, these measures were originally derived from the voice science literature and were adapted for use as suggested by the work of Beckett (1971) and Michel and Wendahl (1971).

Table 6-1 provides a brief operational summary of the measurements and an abbreviation key used in the data tables that follow. The results of these investigations provide some preliminary data regarding the performance of children and adults with normal voices on the measurement battery.

INVESTIGATIONS WITH CHILDREN

Williams (1977) examined 60 elementary school children, 30 of whom were sixth graders, with a mean age of 11 years 9 months, a mean height of 58.3 inches, and a mean weight of 88 pounds. The remaining 30 children were third graders, with a mean age of 8 years 9 months, a mean height of 51.4 inches, and a mean weight of 63.5 pounds.

Respirometric and phonatory measures of vital capacity, phonation time, and phonation volume were obtained. From these three measurements, the other computational measures selected for the battery (Table 6-1) were obtained.

The children were sent singly to the testing room. On arrival, they were weighed and measured for height. They were then instructed to stand up straight and were given instructions on how to exhale into the respirometer to obtain vital capacity measurements, and then how to phonate /u/ into the respirometer for the measurement of phonation volume. Following vital capacity and phonation volume measurements, each child then sustained /a/ at conversational intensity for as long as possible, while being timed with a stopwatch for the phonation time measure. Three trails for each measure were obtained, and the maximum performance on each measure was used in the results.

Tables 6-2 and 6-3 summarize the results of the Williams study by age groups.

Child (1979) investigated 40 fourth grade children with a mean age of 10 years 2 months, a mean height of 55.0 inches, and a mean weight of 76.7 pounds. None of the subjects had had any discernible previous voice problems, nor did they have colds or any similar type of irritations that might have affected their vocal production ability. The same measurement battery used by Williams (1977) was also used in this study. In addition, Child was interested in the number of trials as a variable in the phonation time parameter.

Table 6–1. Descriptive Summary of the Measurements Used in the Investigations

Name	Definition	How Measured	Data Provide/Indicate
Vital capacity (VC)	Maximum volume of air that can be exhaled following maximum inhalation. Expressed in cubic centimeters.	Person exhales maximally into a respirometer after maximum inhalation.	Estimate of amount of air available for production of phonation
Phonation volume (PV)	Maximum volume of air that is used for maximally sustained phonation. Expressed in cubic centimeters.	Person phonates /a/ or /u/ into a respirometer after a maximum inhalation.	Actual phonated volume of air.
Phonation time (PT)	Maximum time an individual can sustain phonation after taking a minimum inhalation. Expressed in seconds.	Person is timed while phonating /a/ after maximal inhalation.	Durational performance measure for sustaining a vowel.
Phonation quotient (PQ)	Ratio of vital capacity and phonation time, providing an estimate of potential air flow. Expressed in cubic centimeters per second.	Computed measurement. Vital capacity/phonation time. $\frac{VC}{PT} = PQ$	Potential air flow; indirect air flow measurement.
Maximum predicted phonation time (MPPT)	Maximum phonation time of an individual as predicted by vital capacity. Expressed in seconds.	Computed measurement, vital capacity/110 × 0.67 male subjects; Vital capacity/110 × 0.59 female subjects (normal adults). (From Yanagihara and von Leden [1967])	Predicted phonation time as suggested by vital capacity.

Table 6-1 (continued).

Name	Definition	How Measured	Data Provide/Indicate
Phonation time ratio (PTR)	Ratio between phonation time and predicted phonation time. Expressed as a decimal value.	Computed measurement. Phonation time/maximum predicted phonation time. $\dfrac{PT}{MPPT}$	Indication of the relationship between predicted and actual phonation time.
Maximum flow rate (MFR)	Rate of air flow during phonation. Expressed in cubic centimeters of air per second.	Computed measurement. Phonation volume/phonation time. $\dfrac{PV}{PT}$	Indirect air flow measured using actual phonated air as measured by phonation volume and actual duration performance.
Vocal velocity index (VVI)	Ratio between maximum air flow and vital capacity during sustained phonation.	Computed measurement. Maximum flow rate/vital capacity. $\dfrac{MFR}{VC}$ (liters) (From Koike and Hirano [1968])	Hypotensive and hypertensive modes of phonation.
Phonation volume vital capacity ratio (PVVR)	Ratio between vital capacity and phonation time. Expressed as a decimal value.	Computed measurement. Phonation volume/vital capacity. $\dfrac{PV}{VC}$	Air consumption ratio between actual phonated air available for phonation and that actually used.

Table 6–2. Adjusted Means and Standard Deviations for the Third Grade and by Sex (Williams, 1977)

Measures	Total (n = 30)		Girls (n = 15)		Boys (n = 15)	
	Mean	SD	Mean	SD	Mean	SD
Height (in.)	51.4	2.8	52.4	3.0	50.3	2.1
Weight (lb.)	63.5	11.0	66.3	11.4	50.8	10.2
VC (cc)	1690.0	340.2	1620.4	329.4	1760.0	347.5
PV (cc)	1541.7	339.4	1480.0	322.8	1603.3	355.2
PT (s)	13.4	.4	13.6	5.2	13.3	2.5
PQ (cc/s)	132.3	41.8	133.3	46.5	131.2	38.2
MPT (s)	10.7	3.1	10.4	3.4	11.0	2.6
PTR (ratio)	1.3	.5	1.4	.6	1.3	.4
MFR (cc/s)	120.6	40.2	120.8	42.8	120.3	38.9
VVI (ratio)	72.6	23.8	76.5	29.3	68.7	16.7

Table 6–3. Adjusted Means and Standard Deviations for the Sixth Grade and by Sex (Williams, 1977)

Measures	Total (n = 30)		Girls (n = 15)		Boys (n = 15)	
	Mean	SD	Mean	SD	Mean	SD
Height (in.)	58.5	3.2	58.6	2.7	58.6	3.7
Weight (lb.)	88.0	17.4	85.3	15.1	90.5	19.4
VC (cc)	2289.6	352.1	2235.7	347.0	2340.0	361.6
PV (cc)	2096.5	356.5	2039.3	328.3	2150.0	384.5
PT (s)	16.9	4.5	15.8	4.1	17.8	4.7
PQ (cc/s)	145.1	.4	148.8	38.6	141.7	47.8
MPT (s)	14.0	2.8	13.3	2.0	14.8	3.2
PTR (ratio)	1.2	.3	1.2	.3	1.3	.4
MFR (cc/s)	134.2	44.1	137.0	41.1	131.5	48.0
VVI (ratio)	59.7	20.8	62.3	22.3	56.7	19.7

The mean and standard deviation for each of the vocal parameters, height and weight, were computed for the male population, the female population, and the total population. Table 6-4 presents the results.

INVESTIGATIONS WITH ADULTS

Inglis (1977) used 50 subjects, 25 female and 25 male, ranging in age from 18 to 25. The subjects had no previous history of laryngeal pathology respiratory disease or hearing loss.

The measurement battery previously described was administered. The mean and standard deviations were computed for each group: female, male, and total sample. The results of the study are listed in Table 6-5.

Taylor (1980) used the same battery to replicate the Inglis study. The study investigated the results from 60 young adults with ages ranging from 18 to 26 years (mean, 23 years).

The mean and standard deviation for the total population, female population, and male population were computed for each of the vocal parameters mentioned in the previous studies. The results of the study are shown in Table 6-6.

With these preliminary data available, clinicians may use the measurement battery to track change in their clients and to have a beginning reference from which to gauge client performance. It should be emphasized that these preliminary performance data should not be interpreted as representing what true normal performance should be, because of the small numbers of subjects and the developmental nature of the measurement battery.

Hammond (1981) reported the use of these measurements in successfully tracking the progress of a 9 year old client with vocal nodules who received VARP therapy. Phonation volume, phonation time, and the air flow measures (maximum flow rate and phonation quotient) appeared to be the most sensitive indicators of client progress in laryngeal function (i.e., reduction in size of the vocal nodules).

The following case report illustrates the potential use of these measures as clinical tracking data for the voice clinician.

A 28 year old woman was referred to the Utah State University Speech-Language and Hearing Center by a laryngologist who described the woman's voice pathology as "hypertrophic laryngitis and Reinke's edema." The client gave an extensive history that was consistent with a hyperfunctional genesis of the problem. She was the mother of seven

Table 6-4. Adjusted Means and Standard Deviations for the Total Population: Grade 4, Elementary Students, Ages 9; 3 to 10; 7 (Child, 1979)

Measures	Total (n = 40)		Girls (n = 20)		Boys (n = 20)	
	Mean	SD	Mean	SD	Mean	SD
Height (in.)	55.00	2.90	55.6	3.30	54.3	2.30
Weight (lb.)	76.70	15.50	80.7	17.40	72.7	12.50
VC (cc)	1997.60	335.20	1859.8	260.10	2135.5	350.60
PV (cc)	1761.30	348.80	1604.0	320.90	1918.5	307.80
PT (s)	17.60	5.10	15.1	4.30	20.2	4.70
PQ (cc/s)	125.80	38.00	133.7	44.60	109.8	25.80
MPT (s)	12.00	2.10	11.0	1.50	13.0	2.10
PTR (ratio)	1.50	.38	1.4	.42	1.6	.32
MFR (cc/s)	160.70	33.30	114.7	39.70	98.6	23.80
VVI (ratio)	54.50	17.70	61.8	19.40	47.1	12.40
PVR (ratio)	.88	.11	.86	.16	.90	.10

Table 6-5. Summary of Means and Standard Deviations for the Population, the Entire Female Population, and the Entire Male Population (Inglis, 1977)

Measures	Total Population		Female Subjects		Male Subjects	
	Mean	SD	Mean	SD	Mean	SD
Age (yr.)	21.7	2.3	20.6	2.0	22.8	2.0
Weight (lb.)	145.0	26.5	126.7	16.1	163.2	21.9
Height (in.)	68.6	3.8	65.7	2.4	71.5	2.4
VC (cc)	4196.0	921.0	3479.2	405.9	4930.0	666.5
PV (cc)	3732.0	832.7	3104.0	465.9	4360.0	588.6
PT (s)	23.8	6.6	22.8	4.1	24.8	8.4
PQ (cc/s)	187.6	61.6	157.2	35.6	217.8	67.7
MPT (s)	25.2	5.9	20.4	2.4	30.0	4.1
PTR (ratio)	1.0	.3	1.1	.3	.8	.3
MFR (cc/s)	166.6	52.3	140.9	34.4	192.3	55.0
VVI (ratio)	40.2	11.1	40.6	8.3	39.9	13.6
PVR (ratio)	.9	.2	.9	.1	.9	.1

Adult population age range: 18–25 years.

Table 6-6. Means and Standard Deviations for the Total Sample Population and by Sex (Taylor, 1980)

Measures	Total Population		Female Subjects		Male Subjects	
	Mean	SD	Mean	SD	Mean	SD
Height (in.)	67.9	3.6	65.1	2.5	70.8	2.1
VC (cc)	4174.8	932.5	3376.3	335.2	4973.3	580.9
PV (cc)	3821.3	940.9	3013.3	379.2	4229.2	554.1
PT (s)	25.5	2.89	22.9	5.8	28.0	8.9
PQ (cc/s)	176.00	56.50	157.0	43.70	195.00	61.40
MPT (s)	28.00	6.50	19.9	3.50	30.30	4.40
PTR (ratio)	1.03	.32	1.1	.34	.92	.29
MFR (cc/s)	161.00	52.70	140.0	40.50	181.00	55.40
VVI (ratio)	40.00	11.20	42.0	10.10	37.00	11.60

Adult population age range: 18-28 years.

children, ages 1 through 9, and observation and report information indicated that she used her voice extensively as the major control stimulus in the home. Yelling, screaming and "hollering" behavior were noted and were supported by reports from her family. Her 8 year old child remarked, "Mom yells at us a lot." The client presented a clinical picture of aphonic instances, occasional diplophonia, breathy production of voice, and observable laryngeal tension accompanied by observable general nervousness. The vocal measures were obtained from the client and were tracked on a monthly basis for the duration of her therapy. Table 6-7 presents her data, which reveal considerable change in the measures from the initial evaluation in April through the month of June. Her therapy program consisted of VARP programming adapted to her individual situation. Progress may be noted dramatically in her improvement during assessment periods, and in June the laryngologist indicated that there was only a small remnant of the pathology on one vocal fold. The reader should note particularly the improvements in phonation time and phonation volume, and the indirect air flow measures (PQ and MFR).

OTHER MEASURES

Eckel and Boone (1981) alluded to the clinical usefulness of objective measurements in monitoring client progress in their discussion of a 19 year

Table 6-7. Data from 28 year old Woman with Hypertrophic Laryngitis and Reinke's Edema: Measurements Over a Course of VARP Intervention

Measures	April	May	June
/s/ max	13 s	15 s	18 s
/z/ max	7 s	10 s	15 s
z/s ratio	.53	.67	.83
VC max	3800 cc	3800 cc	3925 cc
PV max	1850 cc	2200 cc	2650 cc
PV/VC ratio	.49	.58	.67
PT max	8 s	11 s	17 s
MPT max	22.4 s	22.4 s	23.1 s
PQ max	475 cc/s	345.5 cc/s	230.8 cc/s
MFR max	231.2 cc/s	200 cc/s	155.8 cc/s
VVI max	58	52.6	39.9

old university singer with bilateral nodules. Other investigators have similarly investigated various measurement procedures as possible correlates of laryngeal function. Gordon, Morton, and Simpson (1978) measured maximum phonation time for several vowels and reported greatly reduced times in persons with laryngeal pathologies. They also reported increased air flow rates during phonation of these patients. Boone (1977) discussed the use of the s/z ratio as an indicator of vocal fold pathology among voice clients. He reported that vocal folds with pathology appear to function less efficiently, resulting in a decrease in glottal resistance and increased airflow with shortened phonation times. Tait, Michel, and Carpenter (1980) studied children with normal voices, aged 5, 7, and 9, and found that they produced s/z ratios close to 1.0, with /z/ duration being typically slightly longer than the /s/. Eckel and Boone (1981) concluded that the s/z ratio used alone or in conjunction with other measures appeared to be an excellent indicator of poor laryngeal function resulting from glottal margin lesions. Inglis (1977) and Lee (1978) also studied the s/z ratio in their investigations and found them to be sensitive indicators of laryngeal function. Several investigators have reported data on the maximum duration of sustained phonation (phonation time) using sustained vowels (Child, 1979; Coombs, 1976; Kushner and Michel, 1978; Lewis, 1977; Mele, 1981;

Norwood, 1978; Ptacek and Sander, 1963; Wilson, 1979) and have suggested its clinical utility.

Smitheran and Hixon (1981) investigated a clinical method for estimating laryngeal airway resistance during vowel production and suggested that their procedure may be useful in discriminating between persons with normal laryngeal function and those with disordered laryngeal function. The procedure takes advantage of measuring oral pressure and airway opening flow by use of a specially designed utterance that alternates voiceless stop-plosives and voiced vowels. Oral pressure is obtained with an oral catheter, one end being placed in the oral cavity and the other coupled to a differential air pressure transducer. Airway opening flow is channelled through an anesthesia mask covering the mouth and nose. Flow from the mask is sensed by a pneumotachometer, also coupled to a separate air pressure transducer. The resultant conditioned data are recorded on a storage oscilloscope and a thermal recorder. The preliminary data gathered with the system supported the reliability and validity of the method as a way of estimating laryngeal airway resistance during vowel production. The authors cite exploratory clinical evidence to support the sensitivity of the method in detecting differences between persons with and without vocal pathology. This experimental procedure also appears to have great potential for use not only in discriminating between normal and disordered laryngeal functioning but also in the periodic tracking of clinical progress.

The results of these investigations suggest that a variety of noninvasive clinical measures are available to the clinician as potentially valuable sensors of clinical progress. Though many research data remain to be gathered in order to establish their scientific validity, initial investigations have demonstrated their usefulness and relative simplicity and convenience in clinical management.

In addition to these applied clinical techniques, the development of new high technology has created additional research capability to objectify elusive vocal parameters. Davis (1981) discussed techniques for obtaining acoustic measures of voices affected by laryngeal pathology. "These methods use digital computer techniques for voice analysis to extract from the speech signal acoustic measures of vocal function that could serve as clinical aids" (p. 77). Davis (1975, 1979, 1981) suggests that these techniques could produce a profile of acoustic characteristics that would be as useful to the laryngologist and speech-language pathologist as an audiogram is to the audiologist. His findings suggest that it is feasible to use quantifiable acoustic features to distinguish between subjects with and without pathologic voices and to use the analysis for assessing improvement during voice therapy. Davis's profile includes six features: pitch perturbation quotient (PPQ), amplitude perturbation quotient (APQ), pitch amplitude (PA), coefficient of excess (EX), spectral flatness of the inverse filter (SFI), and spectral flatness of the residue signal (SFR). His findings suggested that PPQ, APQ, and EX appeared to offer the most promise for monitoring improvement during voice therapy. Additionally, Gould (1975) and Kojima, Gould, Lambiase, and Isshiki (1980) have suggested additional types of laryngeal analysis procedures using acoustic and physiologic measurements. Perkins's chapter in this volume describes these advances in considerable detail.

Significant new voice analysis instrumentation is now available that undoubtedly will contribute significantly to research and development in the objective measurement of vocal function. Three instruments merit special mention. The Visi-Pitch* can accurately extract cycle to cycle fundamental frequency and can display each cycle in real time. The Voice Identification PM Series Pitch Analyzers[†] are microprocessor controlled and can extract precise acoustic information about both fundamental frequency and intensity. The third instrument meriting special mention is a group of new digital spectrographs*, which allow for detailed spectrum analysis with the newest in high speed components. These high technology instruments have the capability of greatly increasing our basic knowledge about the parameters of the human voice and will provide additional valuable clinical tracking capability to the voice therapy process. A thorough consideration of these potentially significant advances awaits data from ongoing investigations.

The implication of the advances in measurement capability discussed in this chapter is that clinicians can no longer justify a lack of precision on the implied or stated basis that measures of the voice are too difficult to obtain in the clinic. Measurement is a must in the clinical process with any communication disorder, and the area of voice disorders can no longer afford a nonmeasurement mode of operation in clinical management. Voice clinicians must take responsibility for finding and implementing reliable and sensitive clinical measures of vocal function within their clinical settings. The question regarding measurement is no longer "if," but rather "how." Such a consideration can only lead to further advances in the total management of voice problems.

FOOTNOTES

*Kay Elementrics Corporation, 12 Maple Ave., Pine Brook, NJ 07058.
[†]Voice Identification, Inc., P.O. Box 714, Somerville, NJ 08876.

CONCLUSION

In the author's view, the most significant advance in the voice disorders area is the research and development surrounding the measurement of clinical progress. Measurement as a process is basic to full understanding of a phenomenon. If a phenomenon cannot be measured, it cannot be studied, and further, if it cannot be studied precisely, it can never be understood fully. Such is the current status of vocal management. The excitement in participating in the emergence of these measurement procedures is the prospect that in a very short time the voice clinician will be able to validate voice therapy procedures advocated for many years but not validated, and to have an efficient resource available to precisely monitor progress during voice therapy. Moreover, with the development and refinement of these capabilities will come the continued gathering of data, the refining and sorting of effective and ineffective therapy techniques, and, perhaps, the burying forever of those which never did work.

REFERENCES

Aronson, A. *Clinical voice disorders.* (1980). New York: Brian C. Decker.

Beck, M. A. (1976). *The remediation of vocal nodules in school children: A therapeutic program.* Unpublished master's thesis, Utah State University.

Beckett, R. L. (1971). The respirometer as a diagnostic and clinical tool in the speech clinic. *Journal of Speech and Hearing Disorders, 36,* 235, 241.

Beste, L. R. (1971). *Spastic dysphonia—a review of literature and case study.* Unpublished master's thesis, Utah State University.

Boone, D. R. (1977). *The voice and voice therapy* (2nd ed.). Englewood Cliffs, NJ: Prentice-Hall.

Boone, D. R. (1981). Boone Voice Therapy Kit. Gladstone, OR: C. C. Publications.

Brodnitz, F. S. (1971). *Vocal rehabilitation* Rochester, MN: Whiting Press.

Child, D. R. (1979). *Maximum phonation time: Optimum number of trials and normative performance on fourth grade children.* Unpublished master's thesis, Utah State University.

Coachbuilder, D. P. (1972). *Programming vocal exercises for the development of pitch.* Unpublished master's thesis, Utah State University.

Coombs, J. (1976). *The maximum duration of phonation of /a/ in normal and hoarse voiced children.* Unpublished master's thesis, Portland State University.

Cooper, M., and Cooper, M. H. (1977). *Approaches to vocal rehabilitation.* Springfield, IL: Charles C Thomas.

Costello, Janis M. (1977). Programmed instruction. *Journal of Speech and Hearing Disorders, 42,* 3-28.

Davis, S. B. (1975). Preliminary results using inverse filtering of speech for automatic evaluation of laryngeal pathology. *58,* s111 (abstract).

Davis, S. B. (1979). Acoustic characteristics of normal and pathological voices. In N. J. Lass (Ed.), *Speech and language: Advances in basic research and practice* (Vol. 1). New York: Academic Press.

Davis, S. B. (1981). Acoustic characteristics of laryngeal pathology. In J. K. Darby (Ed.), *Speech evaluation in medicine.* New York: Grune & Stratton.

Drudge, M. K. M., and Phillips, B. J. (1976). Shaping behavior in voice therapy. *Journal of Speech and Hearing Disorders, 41,* 398–411.

Eckel, F. C., and Boone, D. R. (1981). The s/z ratio as an indicator of laryngeal pathology. *Journal of Speech and Hearing Disorders, 46,* 147–149.

Filter, M. D. (Ed.) (1982a). *Phonatory voice disorders in children.* Springfield, IL: Charles C Thomas.

Filter, M. D. (1982b). Evaluation of children with phonatory voice disorders: Role of the speech-pathologist. In M. D. Filter (Ed.), *Phonatory voice disorders in children.* Springfield, IL: Charles C Thomas.

Froeschels, E. (1952). Chewing method as therapy: A discussion with some philosophical conclusions. *Archives of Otolaryngology, 56,* 427–434.

Gordon, M. T., Morton, F. M., and Simpson, I. C. (1978). Airflow measurements in diagnosis, assessment and treatment of mechanical dysphonia. *Folia Phoniatrica, 30,* 166–174.

Gould, W. J. (1975). Quantitative assessment of voice function in microlaryngology. *Folia Phoniatrica, 27,* 190, 204.

Greene, M. C. L. (1980). *The voice and its disorders* (4th ed.). Philadelphia: J. B. Lippincott.

Greiner, G. (1973). *A programmed therapy approach to pitch disturbances of the voice.* Unpublished master's thesis, Utah State University.

Hammond, J. (1981). *A precision approach to evaluation and therapy in voice.* Unpublished master's thesis, Utah State University.

Hirano, M., Koike, Y., and von Leden, H. (1968). Maximum phonation time and air usage during phonation. *Folia Phoniatrica, 20,* 185–201.

Hunsaker, J. C. (1974). *Behavior modification and functional voice disorders.* Unpublished master's thesis, Utah State University.

Inglis, J. M. (1977). *Obtaining normative data on vocal parameters in a group of adult speakers.* Unpublished master's thesis, Utah State University.

Isshiki, N. (1964). Regulatory mechanism of voice intensity variation. *Journal of Speech and Hearing Research, 7,* 17–29.

Isshiki, N. (1965). Vocal intensity and air flow rate. *Folia Phoniatrica, 17,* 92–104.

Isshiki, N., Okamura, H., and Morimoto, M. (1967). Maximum phonation time and air flow rate during phonation: Simple clinical tests for vocal function. *Annals of Otology, Rhinology, and Laryngology, 76,* 998–1007.

Isshiki, N., Okamura, H., Tanabe, M., and Morimoto, M. (1969). Differential diagnosis of hoarseness. *Folia Phoniatrica, 21,* 9–19.

Isshiki, N., and von Leden, H. (1964). Hoarseness: Aerodynamic studies. *Archives of Otolaryngology, 80,* 206–213.

Isshiki, N., Yanagihara, N., and Morimoto, M. (1966). Approach to the objective diagnosis of hoarseness. *Folia Phoniatrica, 18,* 393–400.

Iwata, S., and von Leden, H. (1970). Phonation quotient in patients with laryngeal diseases. *Folia Phoniatrica, 22,* 117–128.

Johnson, T. S. (1974). *A precision approach to hyperfunctional voice problems.* Logan, Utah: Utah State University.

Johnson, T. S. (1984). Treatment of vocal abuse in children. In W. H. Perkins (Ed.), *Current therapy of communicative disorders: Voice disorders.* New York: Thieme-Stratton.

Johnson, T. S. (1985). *Vocal abuse reduction program (VARP).* San Diego: College-Hill Press.

Koike, Y. (1968). Vowel amplitude modulations in patients with laryngeal diseases. *Journal of the Acoustical Society of America, 45,* 839–844.

Koike, Y., and Hirano, M. (1968). Significance of vocal velocity index. *Folia Phoniatrica, 20,* 285–296.

Koike, Y., Hirano, M., and von Leden, H. (1967). Vocal initiation: Acoustic and aerodynamic investigations of normal subjects. *Folia Phoniatrica, 19,* 173–182.

Kojima, H., Gould, W. J., Lambiase, A., and Isshiki, N. (1980). Computer analysis of hoarseness. *Acta Otolaryngology, 89,* 547–554.

Kushner, D., and Michel, J. (1978) *Maximum phonation times in 100 adults.* Paper presented to the Annual Convention of the American Speech and Hearing Association, San Francisco.

Laver, J. D. (1968). Voice quality and indexical information. *British Journal of Disordered Communication, 3,* 43–54.

Lee, R. L. (1978). *Phonation and respiratory production in cheerleaders.* Unpublished master's thesis, Utah State University.

Lewis, K. (1977). *The maximum duration of phonation of /a/ in children.* Unpublished master's thesis, Portland State University.

Lubker, J. F. (1979). Acoustic-perceptual methods for evaluation of defective speech. In N. H. Lass (Ed.), *Speech and language: Advances in basic research and practice* (Vol. 1). New York: Academic Press.

Mele, L. (1981). *Maximum phonation time in children four and five years of age.* Unpublished manuscript, James Madison University.

Michel, J. F., and Wendahl, R. (1971). Correlates of voice production. In L. E. Travis (Ed.), *Handbook of speech pathology and audiology.* New York: Appleton-Century-Crofts.

Miller, L. K. (1980). *Principles of everyday behavior analysis.* Monterey, CA: Brooks/Cole.

Moore, G. P. (1977). Have the major issues in voice disorders been answered by research in speech science? A 50 year retrospective. *Journal of Speech and Hearing Disorders, 42,* 152–160.

Moses, P. (1954). *The voice of neurosis.* New York: Grune & Stratton.

Mowrer, D. E. (1982). *Methods of modifying speech behaviors* (2nd ed.). Columbus, OH: Charles E. Merrill.

Murry, T. (1982) Phonation: Remediation. In N. J. Lass, L. V. McReynolds, and J. Northern (Eds.), *Speech, language and hearing: Pathologies of speech and language* (Vol 2). Philadelphia: W. B. Saunders.

Nell, G. W. (1968). An evaluation of behavior therapy in the handling of functional dysphonia in children. *Journal of the South African Logopedic Society, 15,* 14–18.

Norwood, E. D. (1978). *Variability in test-retest of maximum duration of sustained /a/ in children.* Unpublished master's thesis, Portland State University.

Parrish, M. L. (1972). *A therapeutic program for the remediation of vocal nodules in children.* Unpublished master's thesis, Utah State University.

Perkins, W. H. (1971). Vocal function: A behavioral analysis. In L. E. Travis (Ed.), *Handbook of speech pathology and audiology.* New York: Appleton-Century-Crofts.

Pierce, G. L. (1974). *An analysis and reduction of breathiness with accompanying inspiratory speech.* Unpublished master's thesis, Utah State University.

Polow, N., and Kaplan, E. D. (1979). *Symptomatic voice therapy.* Tulsa: Modern Education Corporation.

Ptacek, P. H., and Sander, E. K. (1963). Maximum duration of phonation. *Journal of Speech and Hearing Disorders, 29,* 171–182.

Reed, C. G. (1980). Voice therapy: A need for research. *Journal of Speech and Hearing Disorders, 45,* 157–169.

Rothwell, R. (1974). *A therapeutic program for the remediation of hyperfunctional voice disorders in adults.* Unpublished master's thesis, Utah State University.

Ryan, B. P. (1974). *Programmed therapy for stuttering in children and adults.* Springfield, IL: Charles C Thomas.

Smee, J. S. (1974). *An analysis of contact ulcer reduction using the vocal abuse reduction program and vocal quality program.* Unpublished master's thesis, Utah State University.

Smitheran, J. R., and Hixon, T. J. (1981). A clinical method for estimating laryngeal airway resistance during vowel production. *Journal of Speech and Hearing Disorders, 46,* 138–146.

Tait, N. A., Michel, J. F., and Carpenter, M. A.(1980). Maximum duration of sustained /s/ and /z/ in children. *Journal of Speech and Hearing Disorders, 45,* 239–246.

Taylor, T. J. (1980). *Air flow parameters in college-age individuals.* Unpublished master's thesis, Utah State University.

Thompson, C. G. (1976). *The feasibility of using respirometer measurements as a monitoring agent of laryngeal functioning during vocal nodule rehabilitation.* Unpublished master's thesis, Utah State University.

Vance, S. E. (1976). *A therapeutic approach to an extended length of utterance program for extension and generalization of appropriate vocal quality production.* Unpublished master's thesis, Utah State University.

Williams, K. (1977). *Performances of elementary school aged children on respirometric and phonatory measures.* Unpublished master's thesis, Utah State University.

Williams, S. W. (1979). *A comparative analysis of the Collins P-900 9 liter respirometer and the dropper compact spirometer.* Unpublished master's thesis, Utah State University.

Wilson, D. K. (1979). *Voice problems of children.* Baltimore: Williams & Wilkins.

Wilson, F. B. (1972). The voice disordered child: A descriptive approach. *Language, Speech, and Hearing Services in the Schools, 4,* 14–22.

Wilson, F. B., and Rice, M. (1977). *A programmed approach to voice therapy.* Austin, TX: Learning Concepts.

Yanagihara, N., and Koike, Y. (1967). The regulation of sustained phonation. *Folia Phoniatrica, 19,* 1–18.

Yanagihara, N., Koike, Y., and von Leden, H. (1966). Phonation and respiration. *Folia Phoniatrica, 18,* 323–340.

Yanagihara, N., and von Leden, H. (1967). Respiration and phonation. *Folia Phoniatrica, 19,* 153–166.

PART III
Stuttering

Chapter 7

Treatment of Fluency Disorders: State of the Art

M. N. Hegde

THEORIES AND THERAPIES

It is well known that stuttering is a "disorder of many theories" (Jonas, 1977, p. 7). As such, it is also a disorder of many therapies. It is generally thought that the treatment procedures of a disorder are derived from a theory of that disorder. It must be noted, however, that there are different kinds of theories and only a certain kind can tell the clinician how to treat the disorder. The philosophy of science recognizes two main types of theories: hypothetico-deductive and inductive. The hypothetico-deductive, the classic type, has had some remarkable success in the natural sciences. In order to develop this kind of theory, the researcher first defines some basic terms and then proposes a series of postulates that describe and explain the phenomenon under investigation. Often, these postulates themselves are not directly testable. Therefore, the researcher deduces some theorems from them. These theorems are experimentally tested, and when supported by the results, the theoretical postulates from which they were derived are said to be valid. In essence, deductive theories are predictive models based on logic and mathematics. If the predictions made by the theory are empirically supported, the theory is said to be validated. If not, the theory is appropriately modified or rejected.

The inductive theories, on the other hand, do not start out as predictive models. Instead, they stay close to experimental evidence. While the hypothetico-deductive theory emerges from a logical premise, the inductive theory emerges from data that are experimentally derived, are replicated to some extent, and are known to have a certain degree of generality. The scientist within the deductive framework first suggests a theory, albeit with some evidence, and then sets out a program of research to verify it. The scientist within the inductive framework first performs a series of experiments (and continues to do so) and then lets the results shape theoretic statements.

In the behavioral sciences, Hull's (1951) learning theory illustrates the hypothetico-deductive method, whereas Skinner's (1953, 1969, 1974) experimental analysis of behavior illustrates the inductive method. In the field of learning and conditioning, the Hullian type of deductive theories have not been very successful. Initially, Skinner's main concern was to isolate the controlling variables of behaviors and his theoretical analyses (1969, 1974) came after at least 30 years of experimental research. Skinner rejects theories that are devoid of *demonstrated* empirical relationships but not those based on controlled experimental evidence. Deductive theories have fared better in the natural sciences because of the relatively long tradition of experimental research and the ease with which certain physical and chemical phenomena can be controlled and manipulated. Validated deductive theories are just fine, but it takes a long time to validate them. Meanwhile, scientists and practitioners can get stuck with a theory that may eventually be rejected.

A theory, in its broadest sense, not only describes all aspects of a phenomenon, but also explains why it is taking place by specifying its controlling (independent) variables. By manipulation of the controlling variables, the event can be changed. As can be seen, the clinician needs access to controlling variables of a disorder in order to modify it. It is thus clear that in an applied discipline such as ours, only an inductive theory based on *already demonstrated* controlling variables of events can be of immediate practical significance. Hypothesized but not yet demonstrated cause-effect relationships are of no use to the clinician. Similarly, processes that are presumed to take place in the nervous system but are not manipulable, and fictional psychologic variables such as self-image, provide for neither theoretic rigor nor clinical strategy. As such, experimental research is not restricted to laboratory science. A clinical profession can make no progress without it.

It is both surprising and unfortunate that in the field of stuttering there are hardly any theories that are validated either deductively or inductively. It is surprising because stuttering has been one of the most researched of the speech-language disorders. It is unfortunate because a lack of agreement on the controlling variables of stuttering has led to fruitless theoretic controversies and inefficient therapeutic diversity. History supports the statement that stuttering is a disorder of many pseudo-theories and therapies. This may be largely due to an abundance of nonexperimental research.

From a historical perspective, it cannot be said that effective stuttering therapies have been derived from stuttering theories. Theories and therapies have often been on different courses, resulting in conceptual inconsistencies.

Therapies recommended by many have had very little logical or empirical connection with their own theoretical positions. For example, during the 1930s, when stuttering was explained at the University of Iowa on the basis of disturbed lateral dominance, recommended treatment was often psychologic. As noted by Bloodstein, "It is a curious feature of an essentially neurophysiological breakdown theory that it permits considerable emphasis in therapy on the stutterer's attitudes and adjustments" (1981, p. 345). In more recent years, West and Ansberry (1968) considered stuttering to be an organic disease due to subtle neurologic lesions and atavistic heredity; but when it came to stuttering therapy, they recommended, among other things, that the stutterer's self-confidence be developed (Hegde, 1970).

Many of the current research trends are based on neurophysiologic models of one kind or another. These models postulate that neurophysiologic, neuromotor, or central neural processes, or a combination thereof, are causally involved in stuttering. As yet, no clear cut treatment procedures have been derived from these theoretic positions, although this fact by itself does not necessarily cast doubt on the validity of those hypotheses.

A possible reason why neurophysiologic research has not suggested new or more effective treatments is that, for the most part, this kind of research has not been about the controlling variables of stuttering. It has been about stuttering itself. In other words, the dependent variable (stuttering), not its independent variable(s), has been studied at levels that were inaccessible before. Since by definition, treatment procedures are independent variables the manipulation of which will change the effect, research that focuses almost exclusively on the response properties may not lead to therapeutic tactics.

In the overall scheme of treatment development, neurophysiologic descriptions of stuttering can serve a more useful purpose than theories thereof. Such descriptions tell us about the neurophysiologic events that are a part of stuttering. A knowledge of these events can help us define the treatment targets better, although it does not determine the treatment variables. As long as we heed Perkins's (1981) caution that an integral part of an effect cannot be the cause of the total effect, we will not confuse cause-effect relations and hence will keep treatment targets and procedures separate.

The rest of this chapter concerns various aspects of stuttering treatment. First, we shall look at some treatment procedures whose application seems to have declined over the years. Second, we shall review a recent revival of a therapeutic philosophy concerning attitudinal therapy.

Third, we shall examine major contemporary approaches to stuttering therapy. Fourth, we shall identify elements that are common to several different treatment programs.

NOISE, RHYTHMIC STIMULATION, AND ANXIETY REDUCTION PROCEDURES: YET TO BE PROVED

The scarcity of published reports suggests that the use of such techniques as masking noise, metronome-conditioned speech, and anxiety reduction procedures (involving biofeedback and systematic desensitization) has somewhat declined. The author realizes that statements such as this should be made with a good deal of caution, since stuttering treatment procedures are notorious for their rebirths, and, ipso facto, repeated deaths. Nonetheless, the effectiveness of some of these procedures has not been established, and sophisticated studies are simply lacking.

Noise as a Form of Treatment

Ever since it was found that different levels of auditory masking noise can reduce the frequency of stuttering, attempts have been made to develop treatment procedures based on this finding (Cherry, Sayers, and Marland, 1955; Shane, 1955). Unfortunately, the masking noise procedure always had technical problems. Since the initial masking units were bulky, the treatment was restricted to the clinical situation. Then came the portable electronic models, but they posed the problem of social acceptance. These units required the stutterer to wear double earphones, which tend to evoke undue social attention. The double earphones reduce some hearing acuity for the stutterer and suggest hearing loss to the listener. The most important reason for the decline of masking noise therapy may be its lack of long term effects, however.

There is a general agreement that masking noise of various intensities can reduce stuttering as soon as it is introduced, and perhaps over a short period of time. But the long term effects are a different story. A study by Garber and Martin (1974) has shown that when the masking noise is presented over four to six treatment sessions, there may be no consistent reduction in stuttering frequency across sessions as well as subjects.

The introduction of a voice activated noise unit called the Edinburgh Masker has rekindled some interest in the masking noise procedure (Dewar,

Dewar, and Barnes, 1976). The voice activated unit is technically more sophisticated in that it delivers noise only when the stutterer is talking. Unfortunately, the results of a study by Dewar and colleagues have established neither long term effects nor information on whether the stutterer can be eventually fluent without the masking noise. Further, Ingham, Southwood, and Horsburgh (1981) demonstrated experimentally the wide range of effects (and noneffects) the Edinburgh Masker can have on the stuttering of individual subjects during both oral reading and spontaneous monologue speech. Even if it becomes established that the effects of masking noise do not diminish over time for those subjects who show reliable reductions of stuttering, the procedure may not be acceptable to many stutterers if they have to wear the unit indefinitely.

Rhythmic Stimulation

As a form of stuttering therapy, rhythmic stimulation is both ancient and modern. The most researched signal is auditory, generated by a metronome of either the old desk variety or the modern behind-the-ear electronic model. When the stutterer times his or her syllables or words to the beats of a metronome, there is usually a reduction in stuttering and speech rate. The resulting "fluency" is somewhat deliberate and lacks the normal intonational patterns.

The most promising results with the rhythmic procedure were originally reported by Brady (1971). His Metronome Conditioned Speech retraining procedure was considered effective in 23 stutterers. A followup conducted at 6 to 44 months after therapy showed that 90 per cent of his stutterers had sustained significant improvement. Brady's (1971) promising report prompted a few additional studies, but unfortunately, the results have not been encouraging. Studies by Berman and Brady (1973), Adams and Hotchkiss (1973), Trotter and Silverman (1974), Ost, Gotestam, and Melin (1976), and Silverman (1976), while reporting some positive findings, have actually raised a number of questions about the metronome-conditioned speech. None of these studies have established generalized fluency sustained over a prolonged period of time without equipment. The personal experience of Silverman (1976) suggests that when the unit is used for a long period of time, it may cease to be effective in controlling stuttering.

Anxiety Reduction

In behavior therapy, anxiety reduction procedures such as systematic desensitization and biofeedback have not been very effective. When applied to stuttering, these procedures turn out to be indirect forms of treatment. In anxiety reduction procedures, the focus is on the psychophysiologic state of the speaker, not stuttered speech. In systematic desensitization (also known as reciprocal inhibition), the stutterer's anxiety and fear responses relative to the act of speaking and speaking situations are reduced. This is accomplished by teaching the client deep muscle relaxation and having the person imagine himself or herself speaking in difficult situations. Then, progressively more difficult situations are presented. When this is done repeatedly, the relaxation response is expected to reciprocally inhibit anxiety associated with speech tasks. The assumption has been that if a stutterer's anxiety is eliminated, stuttering will decrease. In biofeedback, various kinds of electronic instruments are used to display information concerning psychophysiologic functions such as muscle tension, blood pressure, and electromyographic activity. By and large, biofeedback as applied to stuttering is also designed to reduce the stutterer's anxiety and muscle tension with the assumption that a relaxed stutterer can speak without stuttering.

Both systematic desensitization and biofeedback seemingly make sense in view of the impression that anxiety and tension are often associated with stuttered speech. Unfortunately, the clinical application of these two procedures has been neither extensive nor very encouraging. Studies on reciprocal inhibition (Boudreau and Jeffrey, 1973; Burgraff, 1974; Moleski and Tosi, 1976; Tyre, Maisto, and Companik, 1973; Yonovitz, Shepherd, and Garrett, 1977), and biofeedback (Guitar, 1975; Hanna, Wilfling, and McNeil, 1975; Lanyon, Barrington, and Newman, 1976) have produced some positive findings, but data on the long term effects are lacking. The use of these two techniques does not appear to be on the increase. As we will see later, more successful techniques teach certain specific responses that lead to nonstuttered speech, and all of these responses are speech-related. Normally, a relaxed neuromuscular state may be a helpful background variable for fluency, but relaxation by itself does not teach the stutterer the skills necessary to produce nonstuttered speech.

A PHILOSOPHIC REVIVAL: ATTITUDINAL THERAPY

A therapeutic philosophy that has staged a sort of comeback relates to stutterers' attitudes and their therapeutic modifications. Historical research on stutterers' attitudes and feelings include two distinct perspectives. An empirical perspective has attempted to describe the kinds of attitudes and feelings the stutterer exhibits (see Bloodstein, 1981, for a review). As can be expected, a speech disorder such as stuttering is bound to have some effect on practically every aspect of the stutterer's life. The person who stutters may evoke unusual reactions from peers, parents, teachers, strangers, and prospective employers. Whether most listeners do indeed react negatively or not, the stutterer is likely to feel that they do. Stuttering can restrict social life and occupational choices. It may alter educational plans and create unpleasant family relationships. Ordinary speaking situations may be traumatic, and the stutterer may learn to avoid them.

Largely because of such personal experience, stutterers may come to entertain a set of beliefs about themselves in relation to their stuttering. The typical set of thoughts stutterers entertain about themselves, when verbalized, is often referred to as "self-image." Stutterers may also feel less confident about themselves because of repeated failures in speaking situations.

Although many clinicians and researchers may believe that for at least some persons stuttering produces personal, emotional, social, and cognitive effects, a controversy arises in regard to the role of these phenomena in the treatment of stuttering. Traditionally, it has been assumed that in order to achieve lasting fluency, attitudes must be changed; if the treatment is designed only to reduce stuttering and increase nonstuttered speech, maladaptive attitudes do not change, and these unchanged attitudes will soon wipe out the temporary and shaky fluency generated by a treatment procedure whose exclusive concern was to modify the stuttering/nonstuttering rates.

How are attitudes, feelings, and self-images changed? Generally, there is more written on the *need* for attitudinal therapy than on its procedures. Fortunately, Gregory (1979) has given some descriptions of procedures by which attitudes are thought to be changed. In essence, the modification of attitudes is attempted mostly at the verbal level. The clinician, assuming the role of a sympathetic listener, encourages stuttering clients to talk freely about feelings, attitudes, and thoughts concerning themselves and their stutterings. In addition, the clinician offers new information on stuttering, and interprets the stutterers' feelings and attitudes so they can understand them better. Finally, the stutterers' verbal expressions of appropriate attitudes and feelings are approved, while inappropriate statements may be disapproved or ignored.

Many treatment procedures that place an emphasis on directly modifying stuttering and/or nonstuttered response rates do not focus on the stutterer's feelings and attitudes. Specifically, procedures based on operant conditioning, and those that are designed to teach certain target behaviors aimed at altering the stutterer's manner of talking (e.g., slowed speech rate) typically do not attempt to manipulate feelings and attitudes (Costello, 1980; Ingham, 1975; Ryan, 1979; Webster, 1979). This has led to the criticism that behavioral treatment of stuttering can generate only limited fluency, which will not be sustained across time or situations (Sheehan, 1979).

Conceptually, attitudinal therapy would be needed only when certain attitudes cause stuttering or when attitudes and stutterings are independent of each other. Unfortunately, there exist virtually no empirical data showing that faulty attitudes exist before the onset of stuttering and hence cause the speech problem. Possibly as a consequence, most experts who advocate attitudinal therapy seem to do so on the assumption that attitudes and stutterings are independent of each other and hence need separate treatment (Erickson, 1969; Guitar, 1976).

The current interest in attitudinal therapy has been stimulated by the reports of Guitar and associates. Initially, Guitar (1976) reported that pretreatment attitudinal measures showed a moderate correlation with treatment outcome, as measured a year later. This report also indicated that pretreatment attitudes were independent of pretreatment stuttering frequency, suggesting that "attitude measures tap an entirely different dimension of stuttering than do counts of stutters and syllables" (Guitar, 1976, p. 598). The next report (Guitar and Bass, 1978) suggested that those stutterers who had "normalized" attitudes at the end of a behavioral (prolonged speech) treatment program were more likely to remain fluent after one year than those whose attitudes had not normalized. These two studies are thought to support the position that attitudes reflect something other than measures of stuttered speech, and that there is a need for attitudinal therapy.

Because of some methodologic and conceptual difficulties, it may be prudent not to conclude that the Guitar (1976) and Guitar and Bass (1978) studies support a need to modify the stutterer's attitudes. Ingham's (1979) critique of the Guitar and Bass paper has pointed out several of these problems and has prompted Guitar (1981) to reanalyze the original data with a more appropriate statistical procedure. On the basis of this reanalysis, Guitar later concluded that "there is not a significant difference in the stuttering frequency between the group that had normalized attitudes after treatment and the group that did not" (1981, p. 440).

A critical examination of research on attitudes and attitudinal therapy raises several questions, the most important being the following: What are attitudes? How are they measured? What are the effects of attitudinal and nonattitudinal therapy?

Traditionally, attitudes are considered to be certain mental states or predispositions to respond in some unspecified ways. In the context of stuttering, attitudes are often defined as either affective and cognitive responses to stimuli (Gregory, 1979) or as "strongly conditioned responses between the subject's stuttered speech and his environment" (Guitar, 1976, p. 598). However, when attitudes are defined as conditioned responses to stimuli, they then become behaviors, not mental states. Such a description negates the distinction between "attitudes" and "behaviors." In essence, the term attitude (as a mental state) may be a misnomer, and if the phenomenon can be described as behavior, then the term is also unnecessary.

If attitudes are certain kinds of behaviors, what kind are they? A potential answer to this question lies in the measurement procedure. Attitudes are typically measured through questionnaires, such as the Iowa Scale of Attitudes Toward Stuttering (Johnson, 1961) or the Erickson S-Scale (Erickson, 1969). In the latter scale, which has been used by several investigators, the stutterer is asked to respond (true or false) to such statements as these: "I would rather not introduce myself to strangers," and "I often feel nervous while talking." Such measures of "attitudes" constitute stutterers' verbal statements concerning their speech and how they feel about their speech performance. From a logical standpoint, such verbal statements and feelings are probably determined by the stutterer's stuttering in the particular situations being questioned.

A recent study by Ulliana and Ingham (1984) demonstrated that modified (S24, Andrews and Cutler, 1974) Erickson Scale responses were not independent of speech and stuttering behaviors. When stutterers were given an opportunity to suggest the basis of their responses to each of the scale items, it became evident that their own speech and stuttering behaviors largely determined the kinds of responses evoked by the questionnaire. Furthermore, actual measures of stuttering in certain scale-identified situations showed that situations associated with "negative attitudes" were also associated with a higher frequency of stutterings than situations associated with "positive attitudes." This led to the conclusion that measures of attitudes, at least on the popular S24 Erickson Scale, were not independent of stuttering.

It is thus evident that attitudinal therapy can hardly be justified on the assumption that stutterings and attitudes are two separate problems of a stutterer. In all likelihood, stutterers' verbal statements and feelings concerning their stuttering ("attitudes") are a direct result of the stuttering itself. In this case, what needs treatment is stuttering, and a successful treatment should eliminate whatever consequences the speech problem generated. Indeed, the results of attitudinal therapy and behavioral treatments that exclude it both support this contention.

Attitudinal therapy is nothing new, although controlled studies on its effects are not many. Broadly speaking, this therapy is not unlike psychotherapy and counseling, which have rarely been effective in reducing stuttering (Van Riper, 1973; Bloodstein, 1981). Long ago, Bryngelson found that a mere reduction of fear of stuttering and negative attitudes had no effect on stuttering frequency (Bloodstein, 1981). Van Riper reported that when he used psychotherapy and counseling aimed at stutterers' feelings and attitudes in the absence of direct procedures, he obtained "the poorest results of any program of therapy" ever employed (1973, p. 216).

An even more crucial question regarding the effectiveness of attitudinal therapy was raised by a study by Martin and Haroldson (1969). They treated one group of stutterers with "information-attitude" therapy and another group with "time-out from speaking." The subjects in both the groups responded to the Iowa Scale of Attitudes Toward Stuttering before and after the treatment. The results were that the time-out was effective in reducing stuttering, but the information-attitude therapy was not. But more importantly, the attitudinal therapy did not make a difference in the pre- and posttreatment scores on the attitudinal scale. In other words, attitudinal therapy may be ineffective not only in reducing stuttering, but also in eliminating negative attitudes.

The effects of behavioral treatments that do not include attitudinal therapy have shed some additional light on the relationship between attitudes and stutterings. The indications are that the degree to which the scores on an attitude scale would reflect "normal attitudes" after treatment is related to the extent of *generalized* fluency. For example, using the S24 Erickson Scale, Andrews and Cutler (1974) showed that a behavioral treatment program resulted in normalized attitudes, but only after stuttering was reduced in several everyday situations. As can be expected, stutterers continue to express negative verbal statements and feelings about situations in which they still stutter.

Additional data indicate that attitudes are effects of stuttering, and what needs treatment is just stuttering. The well known treatment programs of Webster (1979) and Ryan (1979) do not include direct procedures to change attitudes and feelings. Nevertheless, they have reported that as stutterers become more and more fluent, their unfavorable attitudes decrease.

The issue of attitudinal therapy, though an empirical one, has been argued for too long on logical grounds alone. As Webster (1979) has pointed out, "It is incumbent upon those who stress the importance of attitude change procedures to demonstrate the relationship of such procedures to the efficacy of therapeutic practice" (p. 221). It is surprising that the protracted debate on attitude change has not produced a single experimental study with appropriate methodology. Predictive and correlational studies do not produce definitive evidence. Also, it is best to avoid the questionable practice of arguing from negative evidence that might show that certain treatments do not produce lasting fluency. Shortcomings of direct treatment programs do not necessarily justify attitudinal therapy. What is needed is a series of controlled experiments in which attitudinal therapy is employed exclusively to demonstrate its effectiveness in reducing stuttering *and* negative attitudes.

STUTTERING THERAPIES: AN OVERVIEW

In this section, the major stuttering therapies being practiced today will be reviewed. It is recognized that classifying stuttering therapies into well known categories such as traditional versus current or operant versus nonoperant is not always satisfactory or justifiable (Sheehan, 1979). Organizing treatment procedures according to some general and noncontroversial principle can be useful, however. It appears that one such principle is the focus of therapeutic attention. Some techniques seek to modify the *form* of stuttering, not necessarily its frequency. On the other hand, several other techniques are designed to achieve a significant reduction in the frequency of stuttering behaviors. These techniques also seek to establish speech that is considered normal with regard to the parameters of fluency, although this secondary goal has remained somewhat elusive. As will be seen later, systematic studies on the nature of treated and untreated fluency are beginning to be reported.

Modification of the Form of Stuttering

The historical beginnings of the modern treatment of stuttering within the profession of speech-language pathology in the United States are associated with the names of Bryngelson, Johnson, and Van Riper. Bryngelson's initial treatment procedure, Johnson's extensive empirical research, and Van Riper's treatment regimen have created one of the most influential of stuttering therapies. Eventually, Van Riper, over several decades, refined a treatment program and thereby established a certain philosophy and strategy of stuttering therapy. Van Riper's approach is better known than many other approaches, and the sources are readily available (Van Riper, 1973, 1982).

The Van Riper therapy includes both indirect and direct procedures. The indirect procedures are counseling and psychotherapeutic discussions aimed at changing the stutterer's feelings, perceptions, and attitudes. The direct procedures, on the other hand, are concerned with stuttering itself, and their main goal is to modify the *form* of stuttering, not necessarily its frequency. In essence, Van Riper would teach the stutterer what to do when stuttering is expected (preparatory sets), when stuttering has actually begun (pull-outs), and when stuttering has occurred (cancellation). The stutterer's mastery of these skills results in less severe stuttering, or, as Van Riper has often put it, "fluent stuttering."

Two major philosophic assumptions characterize the Van Riperian approach to stuttering therapy. First, the approach, by seeking to modify only the form of stuttering, assumes that fluent speech may not be an appropriate therapeutic target for most stutterers. It is even suggested that the goal of fluent speech may be detrimental because any therapeutic shortcoming can only compound the considerable emotional and attitudinal problems the stutterer typically experiences.

Second, a significant goal of stuttering therapy is to help the stutterer live with the problem. A well adjusted stutterer who stutters with less abnormality is the final goal. Therefore, the stutterer's attitudes must be changed. The stutterer will have to stop avoiding speaking situations, speaking tasks, and stuttering. Instead, stuttering should be allowed to occur while its abnormality and associated negative emotions are controlled. In short, the stutterer should regain self-confidence and self-respect by accepting the realistic therapeutic goal of controlled stuttering.

Reduction in the Frequency of Stuttering

There are several therapy procedures that are non–Van Riperian in their basic assumptions. These procedures assume that fluent speech can and should be the target of stuttering therapy, mere modification of the form of stuttering is not sufficient, and the treatment target should be a significant reduction in stuttering frequency as well as severity. Some of these treatment procedures do not include attitudinal therapy. A few others do, but not necessarily for the purpose of having the stutterer "adjust" to his or her problems.

The argument in favor of the treatment approach seeking to reduce the frequency of stuttering can be summarized as follows. Whether fluency can be a treatment target or not should be treated as an empirical question, and should not be rejected out of hand. The assumption that fluency is unattainable is understandable in the light of disappointing results of historical therapies. It is true that ethical and scientific restraints prevent the clinician from holding out promises that cannot be kept. Nevertheless, scientific progress in the treatment of stuttering can be made only when presumed or demonstrated limits are repeatedly tested. The clinical scientist must operate on the basis that more effective treatment techniques can be developed.

If fluency is considered a possible treatment target for a majority of stutterers, then a mere modification of the form of stuttering is insufficient. A significant reduction in the frequency of stuttering, so that the parameters of fluency fall within normal limits, should be the treatment target. There is some evidence that with additional refinements in generalization procedures and the normalcy of treated fluency, this target is within the reach of many stutterers.

Several treatment programs seek to establish fluent speech in stutterers. A review of these procedures can hardly be exhaustive; only some of the major procedures that characterize the current state of the art can be reviewed here. Even then, only the salient features of selected techniques can be mentioned. Two criteria have guided the selection of procedures for review: some relation to recent advances, and empirical evidence concerning their effectiveness. Different research clinicians have described somewhat different treatment programs, but there seems to be a set of common procedures across several programs (Andrews, Guitar, and Howie, 1980; Andrews and Tanner, 1982; Azrin, Nunn, and Frantz, 1979; Bloodstein, 1975, 1981; Brutten, 1975; Costello, 1975, 1980; Howie, Tanner, and Andrews, 1981; Howie and Woods, 1982; Ingham, 1975; Ingham and Andrews, 1973; Ingham and Packman, 1977; Mowrer, 1975, 1979, 1982; Perkins, 1973a, 1973b; Ryan, 1974, 1979; Ryan and Van Kirk, 1974; Shames and Egolf, 1976; Shames and Florance, 1980; Sheehan, 1979; Webster, 1974; Williams, 1979, 1982, among others). In a later section we shall return to the issue of common elements across treatment programs.

For the most part, the strategy seeking a significant reduction in stuttering was developed within the behavioral framework. Later developments within this strategy were not necessarily restricted to the behavioral paradigm, however. Nevertheless, a non–Van Riperian approach to stuttering treatment owes its existence to the influence of the experimental and applied analyses of behavior.

Behavioral Treatment: Current Status

From the very beginning, behavioral research in stuttering was concerned with the effects of consequences made contingent on various speech behaviors of stutterers. In one strategy, punishing consequences were programmed for stuttering, or disfluencies, whereas in a second strategy, reinforcing consequences were programmed for nonstuttered speech. The first strategy seeks to directly decrease stuttering, while the second strategy seeks to directly increase fluency. These are only procedural differences, because both strategies have the same clinical goal of decreased rate of stuttering and increased rate of fluency (Hegde, 1978). Eventually a third strategy also emerged in which reinforcement and punishment procedures were combined in various proportions.

Punishment of Stuttering

The beginning of the behavioral treatment of stuttering is often associated with the 1958 study of Flanagan, Goldiamond, and Azrin. (For a comprehensive review of the experimental literature related to stuttering as operant behavior, see Costello and Ingham, 1984.) The study by Flanagan and colleagues demonstrated that stuttering can be punished (decreased) as well as reinforced (increased) by contingent consequences. Within the next few years, Goldiamond began to use an operant treatment procedure that used the delayed auditory feedback (Goldiamond, 1965).

Additional clinical procedures based on operant conditioning were somewhat slow to emerge, however. During the 1960s, the operant research on stuttering was firmly established, but it remained mostly experimental. A series of studies conducted by Martin and Siegel and their associates explored the effects of various stimuli delivered contingent on the stutterings and disfluencies of stutterers and normal speakers, respectively (see Siegel, 1970; Martin and Ingham, 1973, for reviews). The initial studies used electric shock as the contingent stimulus. In subsequent studies, the effects of verbal stimuli such as "wrong," time-out from speaking, response cost, and aversive noise were analyzed. The bulk of the evidence of these studies showed that stutterings and disfluencies of stutterers and nonstutterers can be reduced by a variety of consequences, which led to the conclusion that these behaviors were operant responses.

Beyond such a general conclusion, the studies of Martin and Siegel and their associates revealed several problems and complexities, however. Electric shock, which is known to be one of the most powerful of the punishing stimuli proved to be a weak punisher of stuttering. On the average, only 19 per cent of stutterings were reduced by contingent shock.

This was by no means an impressive punishment effect. The verbal stimulus "wrong," on the other hand, was more effective, reducing stuttering by an average of 38 per cent. With nonstuttering speakers, a much greater reduction (60 per cent) in disfluencies was observed when they were instructed not to repeat or interject *and* punished with "wrong."

Additional problems became evident when a later study by Martin, St. Louis, Haroldson, and Hasbrouck (1975) essentially contradicted the long series of earlier investigations. In this study, Martin and colleagues analyzed the effects of continuous shock, which was terminated every time the subject stuttered (negative reinforcement), and response contingent shock (punishment). In the former condition, two of the five adult stutterers stuttered more, just as expected. But the other three subjects did not show a clear cut, consistent increase in stuttering, a finding inconsistent with the negative reinforcement paradigm. In the second condition, only two of the five stutterers showed a decrease in stuttering. In two other subjects, stuttering decreased initially but increased subsequently. The remaining subject's stuttering did not change at all under the shock condition. Martin and colleagues therefore concluded that the results "yield only equivocal support to the notion that stuttering is an operant response class" (1975, p. 489).

Other studies have shown that stuttering, especially part-word repetitions and sound prolongations, either do not change or actually increase when response-contingent shock is presented (Hegde, 1971; Janssen and Brutten, 1973). On the basis of these and other kinds of evidence, Brutten and Shoemaker (1967) have suggested that part-word repetitions and sound prolongations are not operants. On the other hand, a recent study by Costello and Hurst (1981) has suggested that a different form of punishment (time-out) may be more effective in reducing a variety of stuttering topographies, including some considered to be nonoperants by Brutten and Shoemaker (1967).

Although a consistent reduction in stuttering in the laboratory under punishment contingencies may be sufficient ground to suggest that these behaviors are operant, it may not serve as an adequate basis to develop treatment procedures. Long term clinical effects of shock, verbal punishers, and noise have not been established. There is no evidence that this type of punishment leads to lasting fluency. As a result, there are no treatment procedures that exclusively depend on the presentation of aversive stimuli. Somewhat ironically, this is so not because some studies have shown stuttering to increase under shock conditions, but because the magnitude of the demonstrated effect of aversive stimulus presentation has not been of clinical significance in research with adult stutterers.

Another kind of punishment procedure has produced more consistent, and hence less controversial, results. The procedure considered so far involves the *presentation* of known aversive stimuli contingent on stuttering responses. In this other procedure, aversive stimuli are not presented. Instead, positive reinforcers are withdrawn, contingent on response. Time-out (from positive reinforcement) and response cost are the two specific forms of punishment involved in this procedure. In time-out, assumed positive reinforcers are withheld for a brief period, typically 10 seconds, immediately following every stuttering. The subject is not allowed to talk during this period of time-out. This procedure has not only produced more consistent effects on stuttering, but also effects of greater magnitude than the presentation of known aversive stimuli. Several studies indicate that it is possible to generate virtually stutter-free speech with time-out, especially in young stutterers.

Unlike aversive stimulus presentation, time-out has been used as a clinical treatment program. Costello (1975, 1980) has described this procedure in detail along with data on its effectiveness. A stable baseline of stuttering is first established while the client talks and receives the normal kinds of reinforcers from the clinician (attention, smiles, etc.). The treatment is then started. Every stuttering is followed by a 10 second silent period signaled by a "stop" from the clinician. The clinician also avoids eye contact during the time-out period. After the 10 second interval, the clinician re-presents eye contact, smiles, and asks the stutterer to continue. Costello (1975) has found this procedure to be effective in reducing stuttering in three adult stutterers. A notable aspect of the Costello program is that in the latter stages of therapy, the stutterer is asked to remain fluent without the time-out contingency, and the contingency itself is faded out. By the end of the treatment program the stutterers were able to maintain fluency without the treatment contingency. A seven year followup on one of the three clients indicated that the treatment gains were maintained (Costello, 1980). Effectiveness of time-out in obtaining significant reductions in stuttering with adult stutterers has been reported by other investigators as well (Adams and Popelka, 1971; Haroldson, Martin, and Starr, 1968; Martin and Berndt, 1970).

It is possible that the response cost procedure will also prove to be an effective treatment procedure. A study by Halvorson (1971) showed that when each stuttering resulted in the loss of a point on a counter, stuttering frequency decreased. When one of the three subjects could exchange the remaining points for money, there was even a greater reduction in stuttering during the response cost condition. Because of these positive findings, additional research with this procedure seems desirable.

By way of summary, it can be stated that punishment of stuttering with the presentation of aversive stimuli alone has not been a basis of successful treatment strategies. Researchers' interest in this type of punishment has mostly been theoretic (Hegde, 1979). On the other hand, stuttering-contingent withdrawal of positive reinforcers seems to provide a more effective treatment strategy. Evidence suggests that if stuttering is to be punished, time-out and response cost are better alternatives than the presentation of aversive verbal, faradic, and noise stimuli. It must be noted, however, that more research is still needed to establish the long term effects of time-out and response cost. We need more replications and followup data. Also to be noted is that the effects of any punishment procedure, including the presentation of aversive stimuli, can be enhanced by combining it with positive reinforcement for fluency. Indeed, verbal "no" and "wrong" are often presented contingent on stuttering when fluency is positively reinforced. In time-out, too, continuous reinforcement is provided as long as the subject does not stutter.

Reinforcement of Fluency

It is known that most stutterers speak most of their syllables and words without stuttering most of the time, and behavioral technology can decrease as well as increase behaviors. If punishment of stuttering is not very effective, socially undesirable, or tends to generate emotional side effects, then positive reinforcement of nonstuttered utterances can be an attractive alternative. In fact, one of the significant trends in recent years has been to manipulate the parameters of fluency. This has been done both within and outside the behavioral framework. We shall review some of the major procedures of this kind in this section, recognizing that not all of these procedures are explicitly behavioral. They all share one thing in common: the main focus is either the fluent utterance as a *terminal* response, or a series of responses that *result* in nonstuttered speech.

To begin with, attempts were made to positively reinforce fluent utterances as terminal responses. Most of these were case studies with children, which lacked adequate controls and measurement of dependent variables. A review of these studies can be found in Martin and Ingham (1973), and Hegde (1978).

Martin and Siegel (1966) demonstrated in a laboratory study that a combination of punishment of stuttering and reinforcement of fluency can be effective. The effects of the two procedures were confounded in that study, however. Another experimental study in which three adult stutterers were reinforced for speaking fluently was reported by Hegde and Brutten (1977). During the first two (baserate) and the last two (extinction) sessions of this experiment, disfluencies and fluent intervals were measured in the absence of reinforcement. During the middle two experimental sessions, every preselected interval of fluent oral reading was reinforced by the presentation of a dime. When compared to the baserate and the extinction sessions, all three subjects exhibited a greater number of fluent intervals when those intervals were reinforced.

Although it is evident that fluency can be technically reinforced, there are not many studies in which generalized fluency has been established exclusively through reinforcement procedures. It seems that when no attempt is made to alter the speech pattern of the stutterer, reinforcement of stutter-free utterances may not be powerful enough to generate clinically significant (and durable) fluency. This seems to be especially true with the adult stutterer.

Combined Reinforcement and Punishment and Procedures Requiring Altered Speech Patterns

It is thus clear that either the straightforward punishment of stuttering or an exclusive reinforcement of unaltered fluent utterances has not resulted in a comprehensive and successful treatment program for adult stutterers. Procedurally, the two distinct strategies can be combined, however. And this is exactly what is done in several clinical programs.

It is known that concurrent conditioning of reciprocal behaviors is more effective than the exclusive strategies of reinforcement or punishment. However, most of the treatment programs that use both reinforcement and punishment contingencies have also changed the response topography on which those contingencies are placed. Reinforcement is often made contingent not upon the typical stutter-free (fluent) utterance, but upon an *altered pattern* of speech (such as slow or prolonged speech). Treatment programs of this variety have been described by Ingham and Andrews (1973), Ingham (1975), Ingham and Packman (1977), Ryan (1974), Ryan and Van Kirk (1974), Mowrer (1975, 1979, 1982), Howie, Tanner, and Andrews (1981), Webster (1974, 1979) and others. Although there are significant differences across these treatment programs, all of them recognize the importance of the behavioral contingency involving reinforcing consequences programmed for target behaviors and punishing consequences provided for stuttered utterances.

Ingham and Andrews and their associates have conducted a significant series of experiments on stuttering therapy over the past several years. They have analyzed the effects of a variety of treatment procedures with one of the most rigorous measurement procedures ever used in the assessment of stuttering therapy. The treatment program administered by Ingham and Andrews and their associates in Australia is very intensive. In fact, the stutterers are hospitalized for three weeks, during which time they receive 12 hours of daily treatment. Because of their strong commitment to experimental methodology, the treatment program associated with the names of Ingham and Andrews has undergone considerable change over the years. It will not be possible to review all of those changes, although they are interesting from the clinical research viewpoint. (See Ingham, 1984, and Ingham and Lewis, 1978, for reviews, along with Howie, Tanner, and Andrews, 1981).

Initially, a form of rhythmic speech called syllable-timed speech was employed, but it was later abandoned. The authors then added a system of token economy to the prolonged speech method of Curlee and Perkins (1969). In this arrangement, hospitalized stutterers earned tokens by exhibiting nonstuttered speech in order to gain access to various activities, privileges, and necessities. Stuttering exhibited during the several daily assessment sessions resulted in the loss of tokens according to a predetermined schedule. Ingham and Andrews (Ingham, 1975; Ingham and Andrews, 1973) have also used delayed auditory feedback (DAF) to establish prolonged, nonstuttered speech which is eventually shaped back to normal rate. Systematic techniques designed to obtain generalization of treatment effects to the client's natural environment are included. Rate of speech and stuttering frequency are measured throughout the course of treatment and generalization phases.

A recent report describes the current program based on the Ingham and Andrews model as now used by Howie and colleagues (1981). The program is designed to teach Smooth Motion Speech, which is characterized by "slow onset of phonation, continuous airflow and movement of articulators throughout each utterance, and extension of vowels and consonant duration" (Howie et al., 1981, p. 104). The rate is initially slowed to about 50 syllables per minute (SPM). As a result, the speech is virtually stutter-free from the beginning. The normal rate is shaped while the client remains stutter-free in each of the successive stages of this shaping process. Instructions and modeling have replaced the delayed auditory feedback once used to initiate slow speech. Another significant change is that the token economy is no longer used. (See Howie and Woods, 1982, and Ingham, 1983, for an interesting exchange regarding this issue.) Informative feedback and small monetary rewards, which were found to be quite effective, are used to reinforce nonstuttered speech.

The report by Howie and colleagues (1981) offers data on 36 adult stutterers whose speech rate and percentage syllables stuttered were measured on the last day of treatment, after two months in the maintenance phase, and three to nine months after dismissal. Additional data were also offered on 43 stutterers who were followed up 12 to 18 months after treatment. The results showed that virtually all clients stuttered considerably less than before treatment. Varying degrees of relapse were evident in 30 to 60 per cent of the clients, however. Only 50 per cent of the treated clients were fully satisfied with their fluency. Howie and colleagues estimated that with their treatment procedure a stutterer "has a 70% chance of having substantially improved speech and increased speaking confidence 12 months after intensive treatment" (1981, p. 108).

Ryan's well known programmed approach to stuttering modification consists of two major strategies: delayed auditory feedback (DAF) and graduated increase in length and complexity of utterance (GILCU). The treatment of choice is DAF for older or more severely affected stutterers, and GILCU for younger or less severely affected stutterers (Ryan, 1979). Initially, DAF is used to establish slow, prolonged, nonstuttered speech. The amount of DAF is then faded in gradual steps, and the client approaches fluency with normal or near normal speech rate. Successful completion of graduated steps is verbally reinforced, and branching programs to counter failures are specified. An instance of stuttering requires the client to begin the treatment step anew. Both the GILCU and the DAF programs have establishment, transfer, and maintenance phases. Ryan and Van Kirk have offered data on a large number of clients, a majority of whom are reported to have sustained vastly improved fluency in their natural environments (Ryan, 1979).

Mowrer's (1975, 1979, 1982) stuttering treatment program contains several specific steps grouped into establishment, transfer, and maintenance phases. Reinforcing and punishing consequences are programmed for fluency and stuttering, respectively. The program establishes fluency in oral reading and conversational speech, starting with the oral reading of single words. The number of words read is increased gradually until a typical prose selection can be read at a rate of 100 or more words per minute. In most of the early steps, a 95 per cent fluency criterion is required, whereas in the final steps, 98 per cent fluency is expected. The next phase is designed to establish fluency in conversational speech. Transfer and maintenance phases follow. A notable feature of Mowrer's program is that during the initial steps of treatment, 1000 Hz tones are used as stimuli to evoke and time the fluent utterance. The tone stimuli are presented in such a way that the rate is reduced. Eventually, the tone is faded and the rate shaped back to normal. Mowrer (1975) has offered data on 20 stutterers who completed various stages of treatment. Those who were able to complete most of the steps of the program were able to achieve fluency at 99 per cent or better.

A program of research almost exclusively concerned with the direct treatment of stuttering is that of Webster (1974, 1979). Although Webster does not describe his current treatment procedure as being strictly operant, his methodologic and conceptual framework is almost identical to that of operant conditioning and radical behaviorism. Webster analyzes and treats stuttering and speech production strictly at the behavioral level, is highly skeptical of much of the current speculative theorizing, rejects indirect treatment of stuttering through reduction of anxiety or negative attitudes, and has repeatedly urged his colleagues to gather objective, empirical evidence so that we are not "doomed to live forever within the jungle of opinion" (Webster, 1979, p. 221).

Webster's Precision Fluency Shaping Program is another intensive treatment program. About 100 hours of direct treatment are given in a 19 day program. Earlier, Webster had used DAF to establish slow and nonstuttered speech, but later he abandoned it because it did not teach the stutterer those specific behaviors that resulted in fluency. Therefore, Webster began to search for those behaviors that seemed necessary for fluency. His current program consists of teaching stutterers the production of these assumed fluency prerequisites, which include the prolongation of speech sounds (which, ironically, was what he earlier used DAF to achieve), full breath, gentle initiation of phonation, and smooth syllable transitions. He uses an instrument known as the Voice Monitor for teaching appropriate voice onset responses.

Shames and his colleagues have developed and refined an operant therapy procedure aimed at stutter-free speech (Shames and Egolf, 1976; Shames and Florance, 1980). Like several other programs, the recent Shames and Florance program makes use of DAF in the initial phases to slow down the rate of speech and induce stutter-free speech. Continuous phonation throughout the utterance is also required. Establishment of the volitional control of speech is the major goal of the initial phase. In the second phase of treatment, stutterers learn procedures of self-monitoring and self-reinforcement of stutter-free speech. The third phase involves activities designed to promote generalization of treatment effects. In the fourth and the final phase, the stutterer is taught how to maintain stutter-free speech without constant monitoring. A five year followup is also a part of the treatment program. The followup data reported by Shames and Florance (1980) showed that 35 of 37 persons who were examined no longer stuttered, although no quantitative data have been offered. The authors were concerned about the fact that 38 per cent of those who started their treatment terminated it prematurely.

Therapeutic Packages

Another recent trend in stuttering therapy has been to combine several procedures into a therapeutic package. As our review so far suggests, exclusive use of a single technique is a less common practice. Most therapies are a combination of different procedures and targets. A therapeutic package developed by Perkins and his colleagues illustrates this. After obtaining some disappointing results with psychotherapy, Perkins began to analyze and treat stuttering at the behavioral level. He has found the objective behavioral approach to be more effective in reducing stuttering than the subjective and indirect psychotherapeutic approaches (Perkins, 1973a, 1973b, 1979). At the level of the dependent variable (responses), Perkins considers stuttering to be a discoordination of the basic processes involved in the production of speech (Perkins, Bell, Johnson, and Stock, 1979; Perkins, Rudas, Johnson, and Bell, 1976). From a conceptual standpoint, treatment is aimed at teaching the stutterer to use respiratory, phonatory, and articulatory processes in a coordinated manner to produce and maintain fluent speech. Perkins believes that treatment limited to a behavioral establishment of fluency is not complete, however. Psychotherapeutic discussions are also considered of value in coping with persistent use of avoidance tactics.

The initial goal of the Perkins program is to establish slow, nonstuttered oral reading with the help of 250 milliseconds of delayed auditory feedback. Prolongation of syllables is emphasized. In gradual steps, the duration of the delayed auditory feedback is reduced. The next goal is to teach a normal breathflow with easy vocal attacks. Speaking short phrases with sufficient air capacity and continuous airflow is the specific target. Normal prosody is then taught. Next, slow normal speech with DAF is established in conversational speech mode. Establishing a normal speech rate and fading the DAF are the next targets. A clear voice of sufficient loudness is also shaped. Finally, generalization procedures are implemented along with additional counseling (Perkins 1973a, 1973b).

Perkins, Rudas, Johnson, Michael, and Curlee (1974) have published data on the effectiveness of their treatment program. The effects of therapy are evaluated in terms of the number of syllables spoken and stuttered, along with judgments of normalcy of treated fluency, self evaluations, and personality measures. This evaluation has shown that in 17 stutterers, the percentage of syllables stuttered decreased from an average of 9.04 per cent before the treatment to 1.04 per cent at the end of the treatment. Six months later, the rate of stuttering was still only 1.73 per cent. The relapse of stuttering to varying degrees was a problem, however. Only 53 per cent of the treated clients maintained relatively permanent fluency.

Another therapeutic package whose predominant feature is regulated breathing has been described by Azrin and colleagues (1979). The regulated breathing component involves an extended duration of inhalation, an immediate exhalation of some air, and uninterrupted, smooth airflow throughout the utterance. The other components of the program include slightly prolonged vowels, general relaxation training, clear formulation of thoughts before speaking, deliberate pausing at natural junctures, and speaking only a few words at a time. Azrin and colleagues (1979) have reported that the method can eliminate stuttering rapidly. The authors have offered some evidence based upon the clients' own reports on the frequency of stuttering in natural environment. This certainly appears to be a desirable procedure, but its reliability is yet to be established.

There have been several attempts at replicating the results of Azrin and colleagues (1979), but unfortunately the results have not been consistent or supportive (Andrews and Tanner, 1982; Ladouceur, Boudreau, and Theberge, 1981; Poppen, Nunn, and Hook, 1977; Williamson, Epstein, and Coburn, 1981).

SOME CRITICAL RESEARCH NEEDS IN STUTTERING THERAPY

A review of the current status of stuttering therapy suggests that although some significant progress has been made, there still are some critical research needs that the clinicians must be aware of. Issues that need to be researched include the effects of treatment components, both independent and interactive; "normalcy" of treated fluency; and generalization and maintenance of treatment effects.

Effects of Treatment Components

It is evident that regardless of theoretic differences, some components are common to several different treatment programs. To a certain extent, the appearance of therapeutic diversity may be due to differences in the language used to describe the same or similar target behaviors and procedures. It is probable that theoretic biases add certain components to a hypothetical treatment program while subtracting certain other components from it. How much of this addition and subtraction is only in the description of techniques and not in their practice is an interesting question, the answer to which might simultaneously delight and dismay clinicians practicing on the opposite sides of theoretic fences. In any case, the existence of common elements across treatment programs raises some important questions for the clinician. Essentially, we need to find out the relative effects of different treatment components along with their combined and interactive effects. It appears that the descriptions of several of the more successful treatment programs include some form of modified phonation, rate reduction, airflow management, and, to a lesser extent, relaxed movement of the articulators.

Modified phonation seems to have two components: gentle or soft vocal onset and prolongation of speech sounds. The prolonged speech technique has its historical roots (see Ingham, 1984), but the modern interest in it is due mostly to the work of Goldiamond (1965) involving delayed auditory feedback. Currently, prolonged speech is more often induced by clinician instructions and modeling. Much of the recent research on stuttering therapy with adult stutterers has been done with some form of prolonged speech. This has raised the possibility that several other techniques, such as "airflow therapy," "regulated breathing," or "rate control," among others, may be just variations of prolonged speech (Ingham, 1984). Furthermore, in their meta-analysis of stuttering treatment research, Andrews, Guitar, and Howie (1980) have concluded that "treatments based on training a stutterer in prolonged speech and gentle onset techniques are superior to other types of treatment" (p. 305).

A review of recent research on treatment of stuttering suggests that programs based on "pure paradigms" are relatively rare. Most treatment programs include different components, and unfortunately, the name of one of the components often becomes a label for the entire program. Azrin and Nunn's (1977) "regulated breathing" procedure is a case in point. Regulated breathing is but one component in the program, which includes relaxation, "deliberate pauses in speech, thinking out beforehand what you wish to say, adding stress sounds to words, and speaking a few words at a time" (p. 102). Thus, treatment labels (and even descriptions that are often vague) may not necessarily suggest the critical treatment factor in a program.

Equally significant is the possibility that a given treatment component may have effects on other components that are neither described nor measured by the clinical researcher. "Gentle phonatory onset," for example, may affect the rate of speech, which may then become an added and unidentified treatment component. Explicit management of breathstream can induce gentle onset and reduced rate. When the rate is slowed down, the breathing pattern may be changed. Mere simplification of response topography (single words, short phrases) may have an effect on speech rate, breathing patterns, and phonation. Until such possibilities are experimentally ruled out, it may be prudent not to identify the "most effective" treatment component nor to reduce different components to a single one, such as prolonged speech. As Ingham (1984) has pointed out, "it is far from clear which treatment component(s) is necessary either to establish improved speech or to transfer and maintain treatment effects" (p. 372).

What is urgently needed is an experimental analysis of the effects of specific treatment components on the frequency of stuttering. A recent report by Ingham, Montgomery, and Ulliana (1983) is noteworthy in this respect. Their study suggests that it is possible to gain experimental control over a narrowly defined behavior, such as specified durations of phonation. We can expect to understand the treatment process better with this kind of research, in which specific treatment targets are isolated and experimentally manipulated. Once the effects on stuttering of manipulation of different treatment targets are isolated, their interactive effects can be studied. Research on the interaction of different treatment targets and procedures can help combine the most effective treatment components into a single treatment package.

Normalcy of Treated Fluency

A majority of currently effective treatment techniques alter the normal prosodic features of speech. Whether the treatment component is regulated breathing, prolonged speech, gentle onset, or rate reduction, the resulting nonstuttered speech is often deliberate, slow, and devoid of typical intonational patterns. This result is not socially acceptable, and the therapeutic effects may not generalize or last, simply because of this problem. Therefore, concurrent with the establishment of nonstuttered speech, the clinician needs to shape the normal prosodic features.

It seems that before the clinician can shape the normal prosodic features of fluent speech, they must be identified. Research on this issue has barely begun. It is known that listeners can usually distinguish the speech of treated stutterers from that of nonstutterers (Ingham and Packman, 1978; Runyan and Adams, 1978, 1979). Some recent evidence suggests that a critical variable that sets the treated stutterer's speech apart from a nonstutterer's speech may be the rate (Prosek and Runyan, 1983).

It is evident that if the clinical objective is nonstuttered speech that is also not readily distinguished from the speech of normal speakers, shaping of the normal rate should be a part of treatment programs.

Some empirical issues are associated with the need to shape normal rate. Normal rate is a variable phenomenon across individuals. Even a given individual's rate may vary across situations. It is doubtful whether a "norm" can be used in the rate shaping process. It is probably necessary to find out, in replicated series, what speech rates minimize or eliminate discrimination between the speech samples of treated stutterers and normal speakers.

Another potential issue associated with rate control and shaping is whether treated stutterers can sustain both fluency and a rate that cannot be discriminated. Since it seems clear that a discriminated rate is not socially acceptable, clinicians will have to strive towards an indiscriminable ("normal") rate. Nevertheless, whether such an indiscriminable rate is also the one that can help maintain fluency in treated stutterers is yet to be researched.

Finally, the normalcy of treated fluency may not entirely be a function of a certain rate. Rate-related variables are in essence temporal, but there may be factors such as intonational patterns that may not be temporal but topographical. It is possible that in addition to shaping an indiscriminable rate, a certain intonational pattern may also have to be shaped. Clinical experience suggests that when clients begin to increase their rate, their intonational patterns also become indiscriminable. If this is experimentally verified, it would then mean that certain rate and intonational patterns belong to the same response class.

The process of establishing indiscriminable parameters of speech in stutterers may require both measurement procedures and descriptions of those parameters. Martin, Haroldson, and Triden (1984) have demonstrated that "speech naturalness" is a property that can be scaled. However, what temporal and topographical factors are necessary for a judgment of "naturalness" is not clear. As was suggested, rate and intonational patterns are among the most important of the variables. One can systematically manipulate (or shape) these variables independently to see how judgments of "naturalness" are affected.

Generalization and Maintenance of Treatment Effects

Recent advances in the treatment of stuttering suggest that it is possible to induce stutter-free speech patterns within the clinic setting in almost all stutterers, but the treatment effects do not always generalize; and if they do generalize, the effects may not be maintained over time. In the basic research on learning, generalization of conditioned behaviors was considered a natural consequence of stimulus and response similarity. In applied research, however, deficient behaviors that need extensive clinical treatment often do not generalize to the natural environment. This may be so because the treatment environment is unusual (highly discriminated), and the natural environment is still a discriminative stimulus for the deficient behaviors. In any case, only in recent years has the problem of generalization and maintenance been systematically addressed by applied researchers (e.g., Stokes and Baer, 1977).

Most of the researched stuttering treatment programs include a generalization or maintenance phase (Howie, Tanner, and Andrews, 1981; Ingham and Andrews, 1971; Ingham, 1984a; Mowrer, 1975; Perkins, 1973b; Ryan, 1974; Shames and Florance, 1980). There is some evidence, however, that a certain amount of generalization can be obtained in the absence of specific procedures. Most often, such unprogrammed generalization has been observed when child stutterers were treated with stuttering-contingent time-out (see Ingham, 1984a, 1984b, for a review of studies on generalization tactics). Nevertheless, most stutterers, especially adults, need specific procedures to achieve generalized and maintained treatment effects.

There are several methodologic and conceptual issues relative to how generalization is programmed or measured (Ingham, 1984a, 1984b). Generalization typically refers to the occurrence of learned behaviors under various nontreatment conditions and response modes. However, when such generalization is not observed, specific procedures may be applied with the consequence that the resulting response rate may or may not be a product of pure generalization. For instance, the treatment variable may be introduced to the home situation, the parents of a stuttering child may be taught to manage the reinforcement contingencies, or an adult stutterer may be taught some self-management techniques. In situations such as these, it is difficult to determine when the treatment ends and the process of spontaneous generalization begins. Purely from a clinical standpoint, this may be a moot issue, however. If specific procedures are needed to obtain generalized and maintained fluency, they must then be implemented, regardless of whether the effects of such procedures would be considered (technically) to be generalization.

Various tactics for producing generalization have been identified in applied behavioral research (Stokes and Baer, 1977) and in the particular context of stuttering treatment (Ingham, 1984a, 1984b). In principle, generalization and maintenance procedures are designed to minimize discrimination between the stutterer's natural environment and the treatment setting, while simultaneously creating everyday discriminative stimuli for the treated fluency, and to teach self-monitoring skills so that certain treatment variables become ubiquitous.

The first set of techniques is based on the assumption that discrimination prevents generalization and that the client's everyday situations should contain stimuli associated with the target behaviors. Initially, the clinician and the treatment setting become the discriminative stimuli for stutter-free speech while those stimuli are absent in the stutterer's everyday situations. Techniques that minimize discrimination between the clinical setting and the natural environment can simultaneously create new discriminative stimuli for stutter-free speech in nonclinical settings. The latter phases of most treatment programs, for instance, are often loosely structured so that the highly discriminated treatment setting begins to approximate everyday situations. Informal treatment sessions may be held outside the typical clinical setting. The clinician may accompany the stutterer to a store or a restaurant, and manage the treatment contingencies in a subtle manner. Family members or even unfamiliar persons may be invited to the treatment sessions. Treatment may be shifted across response modes such as reading, monologue, and conversational speech. Parents, teachers, siblings, or spouses may be trained to reinforce stutter-free speech in home and school.

The second set of techniques is based on the assumption that if stutterers themselves can manipulate some treatment components, then technically the treatment can be applied in every situation. If the techniques used are effective at all, stutter-free speech should be durable across situations and over time. Those treatment models that teach the stutterer certain skills necessary for stutter-free speech are probably better able to exploit this strategy (Azrin and Nunn, 1977; Perkins, 1973a, 1973b; Webster, 1974). If skills such as reduced rate, gentle phonatory onset, or continuous airflow are part of the treatment program, the stutterer can be taught to maintain them in everyday situations as long as the resulting stutter-free speech is socially acceptable. Within the punishment strategy, there is some evidence that stuttering contingent time-out can be self-administered and thus can help sustain treatment gains (James, 1981; Martin and Haroldson, 1982).

It is evident that a variety of generalization and maintenance strategies have been a part of many treatment programs. Nevertheless, there are very few controlled studies showing that a given strategy was indeed effective. We do not know the relative effects of different strategies. It is possible that some of the generalization strategies are not effective at all. Once again, we need controlled research to document the independent, relative, and interactive effects of generalization and maintenance strategies.

CONCLUDING REMARKS

It is difficult to say that in the recent years some startlingly new or dramatically effective treatment procedures have been developed. Nonetheless, significant progress has been made in the treatment of stuttering. There is now a growing confidence within the profession that a more complete treatment of stuttering is within our reach.

In the judgment of this reviewer, it is better to focus research on stuttering therapy on the *response topography* that needs to be taught or modified, rather than on the procedure with which the targets are accomplished. A reasonably effective technology of behavior change is available, and has been for some time now. We know how to set occasions for responses and arrange consequences that produce desirable changes in those responses. Somewhat ironically, and as Webster (1979) has recognized, what we have been searching for is the target response itself. Much of the research efforts have been concerned with *what* to modify, not *how*. Note that gentle phonation or continuous airflow refer not to independent variables (treatment), but to dependent variables (responses). Additional research with this conceptual framework can be fruitful.

One would hope that in coming years, significant progress can be made in identifying critical treatment variables in relation to specific response properties. Most stuttering therapies are still a conglomeration of treatment variables and response topographies. There is no assurance that all of the described components of a treatment program are always used by the same clinician or replicated by others. We urgently need research that can identify independent, relative, and interactive effects of treatment components and the advantages of focusing on one or more specific response topographies.

Most researchers recognize that we need to develop more effective techniques of generalization and maintenance of treatment effects. Adequate long term followup and measurement of treatment effects through objective procedures are becoming a part of treatment programs. One can expect significant progress in all of these areas. Although there is plenty of room for improvement, research on stuttering therapy is more data based now than ever before, and this might be the most significant of the recent advances.

REFERENCES

Adams, M. R., and Hotchkiss, J. (1973). Some reactions and responses of stutterers to a miniaturized metronome and metronome-conditioning therapy: Three case reports. *Behavior Therapy, 4,* 565–569.

Adams, M. R., and Popelka, G. (1971). The influence of "time-out" on stutterers and their disfluency. *Behavior Therapy, 2,* 334–449.

Andrews, G., and Cutler, J. (1974). Stuttering therapy: The relation between changes in symptom level and attitudes. *Journal of Speech and Hearing Disorders, 39,* 312–319.

Andrews, G., Guitar, B., and Howie, P. (1980). Meta-analysis of the effects of stuttering treatment. *Journal of Speech and Hearing Disorders, 45,* 287–308.

Andrews, G., and Tanner, S. (1982). Stuttering treatment: An attempt to replicate the regulated-breathing method. *Journal of Speech and Hearing Disorders, 42,* 138–140.

Azrin, N. H., and Nunn, R. G. (1977). *Habit control in a day.* New York: Simon and Schuster.

Azrin, N. H., Nunn, R. B., and Frantz, S. E. (1979). Comparison of regulated breathing versus abbreviated desensitization on reported stuttering episodes. *Journal of Speech and Hearing Disorders, 44,* 331–339.

Berman, P. A., and Brady, J. P. (1973). Miniaturized metronomes in the treatment of stuttering: A survey of clinicians' experiences. *Journal of Behavior Therapy and Experimental Psychiatry, 4,* 117–119.

Bloodstein, O. (1975). Stuttering as tension and fragmentation. In J. Eisenson (Ed.), *Stuttering: A second symposium.* New York: Harper and Row.

Bloodstein, O. (1981). *A handbook of stuttering* (3rd ed.). Chicago: National Easter Seal Society.

Boudreau, L. A., and Jeffrey, C. L. (1973). Stuttering treated by desensitization. *Journal of Behavior Therapy and Experimental Psychiatry, 4,* 209–212.

Brady, J. P. (1971). Metronome-conditioned speech retraining for stuttering. *Behavior Therapy, 2,* 129–150.

Brutten, G. J. (1975). Stuttering: Topography, assessment, and behavior change strategies. In J. Eisenson (Ed.), *Stuttering: A second symposium.* New York: Harper and Row.

Brutten, G. J., and Shoemaker, D. J. (1967). *The modification of stuttering.* Englewood Cliffs, NJ: Prentice-Hall.

Burgraff, R. I., (1974). The efficacy of systematic desensitization via imagery as a therapeutic technique with stutterers. *British Journal of Disorders of Communication, 9,* 134–139.

Cherry, C., Sayers, B., and Marland, P. M. (1955). Experiments on the complete supression of stammering. *Nature, 176,* 874–875.

Costello, J. M. (1975). The establishment of fluency with time-out procedures: Three case studies. *Journal of Speech and Hearing Disorders, 40,* 216–231.

Costello, J. M. (1980). Operant conditioning and the treatment of stuttering. In W. H. Perkins (Ed.), Strategies in stuttering therapy. *Seminars in Speech, Language and Hearing, 1,* 311–325. New York: Thieme-Stratton.

Costello, J. M., and Hurst, M. T. (1981). An analysis of the relationship among stuttering behaviors. *Journal of Speech and Hearing Research, 24,* 247–256.

Costello, J. M., and Ingham, R. J. (1984). Stuttering as an operant disorder. In R. Curlee and W. H. Perkins (Eds.), *Nature and treatment of stuttering: New directions.* San Diego: College-Hill Press.

Dewar, A., Dewar, A. D., and Barnes, H. E. (1976). Automatic triggering of auditory feedback masking in stammering and cluttering. *British Journal of Disorders of Communication, 11,* 19–26.

Erickson, R. L. (1969). Assessing communication attitudes among stutterers. *Journal of Speech and Hearing Research, 12,* 711–724.

Curlee, R. F., and Perkins, W. H. (1969). Conversational rate control therapy for stuttering. *Journal of Speech and Hearing Disorders, 34,* 245–250.

Flanagan, B., Goldiamond, I., and Azrin, N. H. (1958). Operant stuttering: The control of stuttering behavior through response-contingent consequences. *Journal of the Experimental Analysis of Behavior, 1,* 173-177.

Garber, S. F., and Martin, R. R. (1974). The effects of white noise on the frequency of stuttering. *Journal of Speech and Hearing Disorders, 17,* 73-79.

Goldiamond, I. (1965). Stuttering and fluency as manipulatable operant response classes. In L. Krasner and L. P. Ullman (Eds.), *Research in behavior modification.* New York: Holt, Rinehart and Winston.

Gregory, H. H. (1979). Controversial issues: Statement and review of literature. In H. H. Gregory (Ed.), *Controversies in stuttering therapy.* Baltimore: University Park Press.

Guitar, B. (1975). Reduction of stuttering frequency using analog electromyographic feedback. *Journal of Speech and Hearing Research, 18,* 672-685.

Guitar, B. (1976). Pretreatment factors associated with the outcome of stuttering therapy. *Journal of Speech and Hearing Research, 19,* 590-600.

Guitar, B. (1981). A correction to "A response to Ingham's critique." *Journal of Speech and Hearing Disorders, 46,* 440.

Guitar, B., and Bass, C. (1978). Stuttering therapy: The relation between attitude change and long-term outcome. *Journal of Speech and Hearing Disorders, 43,* 392-400.

Hanna, R., Wilfling, F., and McNeil, B. (1975). A biofeedback treatment for stuttering. *Journal of Speech and Hearing Disorders, 40,* 270-273.

Haroldson, S. K., Martin, R. R., and Starr, C. (1968). Time-out as a punishment for stuttering. *Journal of Speech and Hearing Research, 11,* 560-566.

Halvorson, J. (1971). The effect on stuttering frequency of pairing punishment (response cost) with reinforcement. *Journal of Speech and Hearing Research, 14,* 356-364.

Hegde, M. N. (1970). Stuttering: A case study in the scientific method. *Journal of the All India Institute of Speech and Hearing, 1,* 104-122.

Hegde, M. N. (1971). The effect of shock on stuttering. *Journal of the All India Institute of Speech and Hearing, 2,* 104-110.

Hegde, M. N. (1978). Fluency and fluency disorders: Their definition, measurement, and modification. *Journal of Fluency Disorders, 3,* 51-71.

Hegde, M. N. (1979). Stuttering as operant behavior. *Journal of Speech and Hearing Research, 22,* 657-671.

Hegde, M. N., and Brutten, G. J., (1977). Reinforcing fluency in stutterers. An experimental study. *Journal of Fluency Disorders, 2,* 21-28.

Howie, P. M., Tanner, S., and Andrews, G. (1981). Short- and long-term outcome in an intensive treatment program for adult stutterers. *Journal of Speech and Hearing Disorders, 46,* 104-109.

Howie, P. M., and Woods, C. L. (1982). Token reinforcement during the instatement and shaping of fluency in the treatment of stuttering. *Journal of Applied Behavior Analysis, 15,* 55-64.

Hull, C. L. (1951). *Essentials of behavior.* New Haven, CT: Yale University Press.

Ingham, R. J. (1975). Operant methodology in stuttering therapy. In J. Eisenson (Ed.), *Stuttering: A second symposium.* New York: Harper and Row.

Ingham, R. J. (1979). Comment on "Stuttering therapy: The relation between attitude change and long-term outcome." *Journal of Speech and Hearing Disorders, 44,* 397-400.

Ingham, R. J. (1983). On token reinforcement and stuttering therapy: Another view on the findings reported by Howie and Woods (1982). *Journal of Applied Behavior Analysis, 16,* 465-470.

Ingham, R. J. (1984a). *Stuttering and behavior therapy: Current status and experimental foundations.* San Diego: College-Hill Press.

Ingham, R. J. (1984b). Generalization and maintenance in the treatment of stuttering. In W. H. Perkins and R. Curlee (Eds.), *Nature and treatment of stuttering: New directions.* San Diego: College-Hill Press.

Ingham, R. J., and Andrews, G. (1971). Stuttering: The quality of fluency after treatment. *Journal of Communication Disorders., 4,* 279–288.

Ingham, R. J., and Andrews, G. (1973). An analysis of a token economy in stuttering therapy. *Journal of Applied Behavior Analysis, 6,* 219–229.

Ingham, R. J., and Lewis, J. I. (1978, Autumn). Behavior therapy and stuttering: And the story grows. *Human Communication,* pp. 125–152.

Ingham, R. J., Montgomery, J., and Ulliana, L. (1983). The effects of manipulating phonation duration on stuttering. *Journal of Speech and Hearing Research, 26,* 579–587.

Ingham, R. J., and Packman, A. (1977). Treatment and generalization effects in an experimental treatment for a stutterer using contingency management and rate control. *Journal of Speech and Hearing Disorders, 42,* 394–407.

Ingham, R. J., and Packman, A. (1978). Perceptual assessment of normalcy of speech following stuttering therapy. *Journal of Speech and Hearing Research, 21,* 63–73.

Ingham, R. J., Southwood, H., and Horsburgh, G. (1981). Some effects of the Edinburgh Masker on stuttering during oral reading and spontaneous speech. *Journal of Fluency Disorders, 6,* 135–154.

James, J. E. (1981). Behavioral self-control of stuttering using time-out from speaking. *Journal of Applied Behavior Analysis, 14,* 25–37.

Janssen, P., and Brutten, J. J., (1973). The differential effects of punishment of oral prolongations. In Y. Lebrun and R. Hoops (Eds.), *Neurolinguistic approaches to stuttering.* The Hague, Netherlands: Mouton.

Johnson, W. (1961). *Stuttering and what you can do about it.* Minneapolis: University of Minnesota Press.

Jonas, G. (1977). *Stuttering: The disorder of many theories.* New York: Farrar, Straus, & Giroux.

Ladouceur, R., Boudreau, L., and Theberge, S. (1981). Awareness training and regulated breathing method in modification of stuttering. *Perceptual and Motor Skills, 53,* 187–194.

Lanyon, R. I., Barrington, C. C., and Newman, A. C. (1976). Modification of stuttering through EMG biofeedback: A preliminary study. *Behavior Therapy, 7,* 96–103.

Martin, R. R., and Berndt, L. A. (1970). The effects of time-out on stuttering in a 12 year old boy. *Exceptional Children, 37,* 303–304.

Martin, R. R., and Haroldson, S. K. (1969). The effects of two treatment procedures on stuttering. *Journal of Communication Disorders, 2,* 115–125.

Martin, R. R., and Haroldson, S. K., (1982). Contingent self-stimulation for stuttering. *Journal of Speech and Hearing Disorders, 47,* 407–413.

Martin, R. R., Haroldson, S. K., and Triden, K. A. (1984). Stuttering and speech naturalness. *Journal of Speech and Hearing Disorders, 49,* 53–58.

Martin, R. R., and Ingham, R. J. (1973). Stuttering. In B. Lahey (Ed.), *The modification of language behavior.* Springfield, IL: Charles C Thomas.

Martin, R. R, and Siegel, G. M. (1966). The effects of simultaneously punishing stuttering and rewarding fluency. *Journal of Speech and Hearing Research, 9,* 466–475.

Martin, R. R., St. Louis, K., Haroldson, S. K., and Hasbrouck, J. (1975). Punishment and negative reinforcement of stuttering using electric shock. *Journal of Speech and Hearing Research, 18,* 478–490.

Moleski, R., and Tosi, D. J. (1976). Comparative psychotherapy: Rational emotive therapy versus systematic desensitization in the treatment of stuttering. *Journal of Consulting and Clinical Psychology, 44,* 309-311.

Mowrer, D. E. (1975). An instructional program to increase fluent speech of stutterers. *Journal of Fluency Disorders, 1,* 25-35.

Mowrer, D. E. (1979). *A program to establish fluent speech.* Columbus, OH: Charles E. Merrill.

Mowrer, D. E. (1982). Treatment procedures for stutterers. In D. E. Mowrer and J. L. Case, *Clinical management of speech disorders.* Rockville, MD: Aspen.

Ost, L. G., Gotestam, K. G., and Melin, L. A. (1976). A controlled study of two behavioral methods in the treatment of stuttering. *Behavior Therapy, 7,* 587-592.

Perkins, W. H. (1973a). Replacement of stuttering with normal speech: I. Rationale. *Journal of Speech and Hearing Disorders, 38,* 283-294.

Perkins, W. H. (1973b). Replacement of stuttering with normal speech: II. Clinical procedures. *Journal of Speech and Hearing Disorders, 38,* 295-303.

Perkins, W. H. (1979). From psychoanalysis to discoordination. In H. H. Gregory (Ed.), *Controversies about stuttering therapy.* Baltimore: University Park Press.

Perkins, W. H. (1981). Implications of scientific research for treatment of stuttering: A lecture. *Journal of Fluency Disorders, 6,* 155-162.

Perkins, W. H., Bell, J., Johnson, L., and Stocks, J. (1979). Phone rate and the effective planning time hypothesis of stuttering. *Journal of Speech and Hearing Research, 22,* 747-755.

Perkins, W. H., Rudas, J., Johnson, L., and Bell, J. (1976). Stuttering: Discoordination of phonation with articulation and respiration. *Journal of Speech and Hearing Research, 19,* 509-522.

Perkins, W. H., Rudas, J., Johnson, L., Michael, W. B., and Curlee, R. F. (1974). Replacement of stuttering with normal speech: III. Clinical effectiveness. *Journal of Speech and Hearing Disorders, 39,* 416-428.

Poppen, R., Nunn, R. G., and Hook, S. (1977). Effects of several therapies on stuttering in a single case. *Journal of Fluency Disorders, 2,* 35-44.

Prosek, R. A., and Runyan, C. M. (1983). Effects of segment and pause manipulations on the identification of treated stutterers. *Journal of Speech and Hearing Research, 26,* 510-516.

Runyan, C. M., and Adams, M. R. (1978). Perceptual study of the speech of "successfully therapeutized" stutterers. *Journal of Fluency Disorders, 3,* 25-39.

Runyan, C. M., and Adams, M. R. (1979). Unsophisticated judges' perceptual evaluation of the speech of "successfully treated" stutterers. *Journal of Fluency Disorders, 4,* 29-38.

Ryan, B. P. (1974). *Programmed therapy for stuttering in children and adults.* Springfield, IL: Charles C Thomas.

Ryan, B. P. (1979). Stuttering therapy in a framework of operant conditioning and programmed learning. In H. H. Gregory (Ed.), *Controversies about stuttering therapy.* Baltimore: University Park Press.

Ryan, B. P., and Van Kirk, B. (1974). The establishment, transfer, and maintenance of fluent speech in 50 stutterers using delayed auditory feedback and operant procedures. *Journal of Speech and Hearing Disorders, 39,* 3-10.

Shames, G. H., and Egolf, D. B. (1976). *Operant conditioning and the management of stuttering.* Englewood Cliffs, NJ: Prentice-Hall.

Shames, G. H., and Florance, C. L. (1980). *Stutter-free speech: A goal for therapy.* Columbus, OH: Charles E. Merrill.

Shane, M. L. S. (1955). Effects on stuttering of alteration in auditory feedback. In W. Johnson and R. R. Leutenegger (Eds.), *Stuttering in children and adults.* Minneapolis: University of Minnesota Press.

Sheehan, J. G. (1979). Current issues on stuttering and recovery. In H. H. Gregory (Ed.), *Controversies about stuttering therapy.* Baltimore: University Park Press.

Siegel, G. M. (1970). Punishment, stuttering, and disfluency. *Journal of Speech and Hearing Research, 13,* 677–714.

Silverman, F. H. (1976). Long-term impact of a miniaturized metronome on stuttering: An interim report. *Perceptual and Motor Skills, 42,* 13–22.

Skinner, B. F. (1953). *Science and human behavior.* New York: Macmillan.

Skinner, B. F. (1969). *Contingencies of reinforcement: A theoretical analysis.* New York. Appleton-Century-Crofts.

Skinner, B. F. (1974). *About behaviorism.* New York: Vintage Books.

Stokes, T. F., and Baer, D. M. (1977). An implicit technology of generalization. *Journal of Applied Behavior Analysis, 10,* 349–367.

Trotter, W. D., and Silverman, F. H. (1974). Does the effect of spacing speech with a miniaturized metronome on stuttering wear off? *Perceptual and Motor Skills, 39,* 429–430.

Tyre, T. E., Maisto, S. A., and Companik, P. J. (1973). The use of systematic desensitization in the treatment of chronic stuttering behavior. *Journal of Speech and Hearing Disorders, 38,* 514–519.

Ulliana, L., and Ingham, R. J. (1984). Behavioral and nonbehavioral variables in the measurement of stutterers' communication attitudes. *Journal of Speech and Hearing Disorders, 49,* 83–93.

Van Riper, C. (1973). *The treatment of stuttering.* Englewood Cliffs, NJ: Prentice-Hall.

Van Riper, C. (1982). *The nature of stuttering* (2nd ed.). Englewood Cliffs, NJ: Prentice-Hall.

Webster, R. L. (1974). A behavioral analysis of stuttering: Treatment and theory. In K. S. Calhoun, H. E. Adams, and K. M. Mitchell (Eds.), *Innovative treatment methods in psychotherapy.* New York: John Wiley & Sons.

Webster, R. L. (1979). Empirical considerations regarding stuttering therapy. In H. H. Gregory (Ed.), *Controversies about stuttering therapy.* Baltimore: University Park Press.

West, R., and Ansberry, M. (1968). *The rehabilitation of speech* (4th ed.). New York: Harper & Row.

Williams, D. E. (1979). A perspective on approaches to stuttering therapy. In H. H. Gregory (Ed.), *Controversies about stuttering therapy.* Baltimore: University Park Press.

Williams, D. E. (1982). Stuttering therapy: Where are we going—and why? *Journal of Fluency Disorders, 7,* 159–170.

Williamson, D. A., Epstein, L. H., and Coburn, C. (1981). Multiple baseline analysis of the regulated breathing procedure for the treatment of stuttering. *Journal of Fluency Disorders, 6,* 327–339.

Yonovitz, A., Shepherd, W. T., and Garrett, S. (1977). Hierarchical stimulation: Two case studies of stuttering modification using systematic desensitization. *Journal of Fluency Disorders, 2,* 21–28.

Chapter 8

Stuttering Treatment Outcome Evaluation

Roger J. Ingham and
Janis M. Costello[1]

Although researchers in stuttering find few areas of agreement, it would seem that today all agree about the importance of systematic measurement in the evaluation of stuttering treatment outcomes. And they would probably agree that over the past decade the management and evaluation of stuttering therapy has been improved by increasing use of measurement methodology. Much of the methodology that has begun to emerge in reports on stuttering therapy is almost wholly attributable to the pervasive influence of behavior therapy principles on stuttering treatment research (Costello, 1982; Ingham, 1984). What researchers still do not agree upon, however, would appear to be the certainty with which current measurement methods adequately account for the constructs implicated in the notion of therapy success or failure. Further, there is no evidence that the measurement methodology described in stuttering research reports has yet invaded the realm of clinical practice (Costello, 1979). The general purpose of this chapter, therefore, will be to offer some considerations on the problems of stuttering treatment outcome evaluation. These considerations will be in two parts: (1) a review of the principal issues in stuttering treatment evaluation, and (2) derivation of a viable clinical format that will assist clinicians and researchers to identify effects of treatment. Both parts will endeavor to identify some of the more important recent developments in the evaluation of stuttering treatment outcome.

[1]This chapter was prepared while Dr. Costello was Foundation Fellow at Cumberland College of Health Sciences, Sydney. It is reprinted from *Speech Disorders in Children: Recent Advances* (College-Hill Press, 1984) because of its relevance to the design of measurement procedures for treatment of adults as well as of children with speech disorders.

STUTTERING TREATMENT EVALUATION ISSUES

The clinical validity of the measurement and treatment evaluation strategies used in stuttering treatment reports continues to concern researchers and clinicians alike (Gregory, 1978; Sheehan, 1980). Much of this concern can be traced to the absence of agreed upon criteria for evaluating therapy. Some attempts have been made to resolve this problem (Andrews and Ingham, 1972; Ingham, 1981; Ryan, 1974; Silverman, 1981), but none has produced commonly accepted methods for determining the clinical merit of stuttering therapy. Some of the issues that need to be resolved before acceptance is likely were recently summarized by Bloodstein (1981, pp. 386–390). He presented 11 criteria that he believes need to be considered when evaluating stuttering therapy. In what follows, these criteria will be presented (mainly in abridged form) and reviewed for their contribution to the search for clinically suitable measurement methods.[2] This will also provide a useful vehicle for reviewing some recent developments in therapy outcome evaluation.

> *1. The method must be shown to be effective with an ample and representative group of stutterers. The single-subject design has a place in scientific research. It has been widely misused, however, in the area of research on stuttering therapy, where most single cases written up for publication are apparently chosen for the precise reason that they were successes. This practice produces a distorted picture. In the end we learn little from it beyond what we already know—that somewhere, at sometime almost any therapy can achieve a remarkable result for some stutterers.*

This is not only a criterion, but a recommendation that therapy evaluation should not depend on single-subject research. This is an important recommendation since it challenges the worth of single-subject therapy research designs. Actually the point at issue is the external validity of these designs. Single-subject research designs entered therapy research for a variety of reasons; foremost was the failure of group designs to identify critical aspects of the clinical process (Hersen and Barlow, 1976). Since group trends usually fail to reflect individual treatment response patterns, they also fail to discern the treatment's differential effects on certain individuals and, hence, themselves do not answer Bloodstein's first criterion. Quite obviously, single-subject studies can only show that a treatment has produced some profitable (or unprofitable) results for some stutterers; but that is far from a trivial finding, particularly if the study is internally valid and clearly specifies the treatment's effects. Furthermore, when such findings are replicated on additional subjects, then they not only increase the generality of the findings as Bloodstein would wish, but also strengthen our knowledge about a treatment and highlight relevant considerations for the design of subsequent group studies.

Regarding the concern about reporting only successful treatments, it is worth noting that this tradition probably permeates group research as much as single-subject research.

In the continuing struggle to find reliable treatments, there is increasing evidence that carefully managed time-series investigations are markedly improving clinical knowledge. Bloodstein's claim that a method must be effective across "representative" stutterers may, unwittingly, subscribe to the "uniformity assumption myth" (Kiesler, 1966)—the notion that there should be a uniform treatment suitable for a uniform client. Even treatment techniques promoted as useful for most stutterers, notably the prolonged speech procedures (Andrews, Guitar, and Howie, 1980), have benefited from controlled single-subject investigations (Ingham, 1984).

> *2. Results must be demonstrated by objective measures of speech behavior such as frequency of stuttering or rate of speech, and by judges' ratings of severity. Such measurements should be made before, during, and after treatment by observers other than the experimenters themselves or without knowledge that might influence their judgment, and due account must be taken of the observers' reliability.*

There are two aspects to this criterion: the types of measures and their reliability. The first refers mainly to the construct validity of measures currently used to assess stuttering behavior. Frequency counts of stuttering and, to a lesser extent, ratings of stuttering severity have become almost *the* descriptive datum for this disorder. Significantly, Bloodstein recommends counts of stutterings, rather than measures of *disfluencies* or *dysfluencies*. Also of interest is the absence of reference to different disfluency categories, a method of measuring stuttering that seems to have faded in its use in treatment. Severity ratings present a number of problems, mainly because there is no agreed-upon method for rating severity. The principal purpose of severity rating during treatment is to ensure that frequency reduction is not offset by worsening severity. One common method for determining severity is to measure the duration of individual moments of stuttering (Costello, 1981; Costello and Ingham, 1984). The difficulty with this measure is that it, too, may lack construct validity, for duration may not be the feature that clinicians or clients regard as measuring stuttering's severity. Speech rate measures, though essential to show that treatment benefits are not simply due to reduced rate, are questionable for similar reasons. At best, syllables per minute (Andrews and Ingham, 1972) or articulation rates scores (Perkins, 1975) only broadly indicate whether the subject is speaking unnaturally fast or slow. And for this reason, there may also be merit in supplementing this measure with perceptual judgments of the naturalness of the subject's speech (see below).

The importance of observer reliability is seemingly self-evident—yet that does not seem to be true for many researchers. A staggering number of treatment reports and experimental studies fail to report relevant reliability data (Ingham, 1984)—a fact that destroys the credibility of much of the current treatment literature. Even when reliability data are provided, they are rarely reported in a way that makes it possible to determine whether a study's reported data trends are also reliable (Hawkins and Dotson, 1975; McReynolds and Kearns, 1983).

One other issue concerns the methods used to obtain stuttering counts and speech rate. There is now a growing body of evidence that clinicians can capably count both of these variables "on line" and reliably (Ingham, 1984).

3. Reports of therapeutic success must be based on repeated evaluations and adequate samples of speech. The great variability of stuttering from time to time and under different conditions is liable to result in assessments that are unrepresentative.

This criterion is simple to justify, but less simple to prescribe. It is unclear how frequently such evaluations should be made, or what represents adequate samples of speech. Repeated evaluation helps determine whether the variability within and between speaking situations has been unambiguously and significantly modified by treatment. This means that the duration of evaluation cannot always be standardized across individuals—a source of difficulty for the use of group designs in therapy research. The same issue applies to sample size, although there is increasing acceptance of a method used by Ryan (1971, 1974)—that is, 5-minute samples of conversation, monologue, and oral reading. However, the sufficiency and representativeness of this, or any other arbitrarily determined sampling interval, is currently undocumented.

One attempt to derive a methodology that prescribes minimal frequency and sample size parameters will be outlined below. But this attempt is also hindered by the impoverished amount of research on stuttering variability across situations—a surprising circumstance in view of developments in recording technology. The problems involved in recording stuttering in "natural" circumstances have also received insufficient attention (Ingham, 1981). However, the advent of portable microcassette recorders should make it possible to obtain adequate speech samples in representative speaking situations.

The method of choosing "representative" speaking situations has also received very little attention in the treatment literature. One obvious method is to derive these situations from speaking log books prepared by the subject in advance of the treatment study; this would help identify situations that can be regularly used for assessment.

Most treatment research presumes that stuttering variability is largely affected by situational factors. Those may not be the only factors involved. Another feature of variability can be a tendency for time factors to influence variability (Ingham, 1981). The duration of time the subject spends speaking in certain situations, or even the time of day assessments are made, might be worthy areas of investigation.

4. Improvement must be shown to carry over to speaking situations outside the clinical setting.

This is much related to Criterion 3. Most clinicians are aware that vast differences may occur between clinic and extraclinic speech performance, but evidence showing this difference is surprisingly small. Studies by Ingham and Packman (1977), Resick, Wendiggensen, Ames, and Meyer (1978), and Ingham (1982a) go some way towards illustrating this criterion's importance.

Another interesting consideration is the boundary of the "clinical setting." The mere presence of a tape recorder or an assessor in the subject's nonclinic setting may evoke clinic-related speech performance (Ingham, 1981). For example, subjects may be assessed via telephone conversations from home or elsewhere, but the accompanying "assessment variables" may make these telephone conversations atypical (see Ingham, 1981, 1982a). The only available solution to this problem would seem to be some form of occasional covert assessment.

5. The stability of the results must be demonstrated by long-term follow-up investigations. Any number of methods for

*making stuttering disappear have been known for many years:
the great and persistent problem of stuttering therapy is how
to keep the stutterer from relapsing. Relatively little is known
about the subject of relapse.*

Long-term therapy investigations are becoming more common, despite
their technical and conceptual difficulties; not the least of these is the length
of time needed to prove that treatment has produced a durable
improvement. Some of the issues associated with maintenance of treatment
effects have been discussed elsewhere (Ingham, 1981) and will be taken up
again later in this chapter.

Bloodstein (1981) suggests that "perhaps eighteen months to two years
is the shortest interval after which most experienced clinicians would not
feel unduly optimistic in hoping that the improvement was lasting" (p. 387).
But their optimism should be tempered by information on what has
transpired in that period. Many current treatment programs incorporate
strategies for preventing relapse. These include speech practice, routine clinic
visits, and continuing interaction with previously treated patients. These
may be useful and even crucial techniques for sustaining improvement, but
they may also confound the most clinically desirable effect—sustained
improvement with the same level of attention to speech that is used by
normal speakers. That is not to deny the advantages of "aided"
maintenance; it simply suggests that clinicians should recognize that there
are different types of sustained improvement. Needless to say, this topic
is in dire need of investigation.

Increasing attention is being devoted to both the measurement and
management of maintenance (Boberg, 1981). There may be some value in
"booster" treatments, and in treatment schedules designed to sustain
treatment gains for increasingly longer intervals. Another interesting area
of treatment research concerns the use of self-management techniques.
There are also numerous suggested approaches to maintenance that need
investigation (Boberg, Howie, and Woods, 1979; Hanna and Owen, 1977;
Ingham, 1981; Shames, 1981). These mainly include self-help groups, regular
speech practice schedules, and the assistance of "significant others." A large
number of other, ostensibly useful, approaches have been reviewed by
Stokes and Baer (1977).

One aspect of relapse that has attracted attention is the stutterer's
attitude towards communication at the end of treatment. The problem of
devising valid measures of attitudes and the shaky foundations of research
claiming that poor communication attitudes influence long-term outcome
are current concerns (Guitar, 1979, 1981; Guitar and Bass, 1978; Ingham,
1979, 1981; Ulliana and Ingham, 1984). Nevertheless, it is highly likely that

persons who show little interest in sustaining speech practice or fulfilling treatment requirements will be strong candidates for posttreatment relapse. The complex factors that enjoin patients to seek treatment, wait lengthy periods for treatment to begin, and then complete its often demanding requirements deserve much more research attention. It may well emerge that these are among the most important variables in the success, or otherwise, of the treatment process.

> 6. *Suitable control groups or control conditions must be used to show that reductions in stuttering are the result of treatment.*

This criterion highlights the need for treatment designs that overcome threats to their internal validity. The advantage of the within-subject time-series designs (Hersen and Barlow, 1976) is that the effect of most nontreatment-related variables can be identified by the judicious choice of a baserate(s) duration and measurement conditions. The difficulty is to be certain that all validity threats have been controlled before, during, or even after treatment. For instance, one important nontreatment factor that is rarely controlled is the amount and nature of influence that the client is able to exert over stuttering frequency or severity prior to treatment. Certainly a treatment's effects should be independent of the extent or duration of such factors.

Group designs as a control procedure can only partially avoid some of the problems of assessing treatment effects because, as was previously mentioned, most fail to identify individual treatment responses. One compromise is a multiple baseline across subjects design wherein treatment is introduced for each subject following nontreatment baselines of differing lengths. Another difficulty with group designs is the choice of an appropriate control group. The best designed group studies presume that roughly matched group mean stuttering frequency, group mean speech rate, and perhaps age and sex, will ensure that the groups have potentially equivalent reactions to the treatment condition. There are literally no data that justify this assumption of uniformity. Even less defensible is the notion that meaningful findings can be derived by merging the differences between subject groups, treatment management techniques, measurement quality, assessment procedures, and treatment time from different therapy studies; but such are the assumptions beneath the use of the "meta-analysis" (Smith and Glass, 1977) technique that Andrews, Guitar, and Howie (1980) used to draw comparisons between different stuttering treatment techniques.

The inherent weakness of meta-analysis for evaluating the effects of a stuttering therapy should be almost self-evident, but it is clearly revealed by examining the foundations of one of the main conclusions reached by

Andrews and colleagues. They concluded "that treatments based on training a stutterer in prolonged speech and gentle onset techniques are superior to other types of treatment" (p. 305). While there is evidence to indicate that prolonged speech treatments are indeed successful for many stutterers, the basis for this claim hinges on an investigation that virtually excluded reference to certain treatment techniques and relied upon extremely questionable posttreatment data from others. By necessity, the meta-analysis technique cannot deal with single-subject studies and so almost all reports on response contingent procedures were excluded from their comparison. (The exception was a study by Martin and Haroldson [1969] which was not designed to evaluate therapy outcome). Also, out of the 12 "prolonged speech" studies included for investigation only two reported using beyond-clinic data, and one of these used an extensive uncontrolled maintenance program in the interval when outcome data were collected (Ingham, 1984). It is little wonder that Eysenck (1978) described this method's concern for data quantity rather than quality as an "exercise in mega-silliness" (p. 517), a concern echoed by Sheehan (1980).

Along with suitable designs for discerning stuttering treatment effects there is also a need for clinically viable designs that determine when treatments are impotent, or are no longer needed because their effects have generalized. These phenomena have been identified in some studies through the use of within-session ABA designs, such as that reported by Costello (1975), or multiple baselines (Martin, Kuhl, and Haroldson, 1972). There is also a need to determine the time required to decide when treatment is *not* effective or, conversely, the changes in performance that indicate clinically significant treatment effects.

7. The subjects' speech must sound natural and spontaneous to listeners, and the subjects must be free from the need to monitor their speech.

This criterion has grown in importance in recent years because of therapies that rely on changing the client's speech pattern. Some investigators have measured naturalness by using listeners to rate speech samples either for normalcy or naturalness (Jones and Azrin, 1969; Perkins, Rudas, Johnson, Michael, and Curlee, 1974). Others have tested whether listeners are able to distinguish the stutterer's posttreatment speech from speech samples of normally fluent speakers (Ingham and Packman, 1978; Runyan and Adams, 1978, 1979). Another approach measures aspects of speech, such as vowel duration or rate, in order to relate the subject's speech to normal speech (Metz, Onufrak, and Ogburn, 1979). A different approach to this task is emerging from research by Martin (1981; Martin, Haroldson, and Triden, 1984), who found that listeners could rate short speech samples for naturalness on a 9-point scale with high levels of reliability. In consequence, Martin and Ingham are investigating the effects on stuttering and speech quality of feeding back to subjects every 30 seconds a listener's speech naturalness rating of the subject's speech. Preliminary results show that clinicians perform this task with high reliability, and that for some stutterers, providing on-line feedback regarding the naturalness of their speech may positively influence their observed speech quality. Similar endeavors have not been made to measure for "spontaneity" but, in principle, there is no reason why listener judgments could not be used for the same purpose.

Regarding the issue of monitoring, Shames and Florance (1980) reported measuring "monitored" and "unmonitored" speech during their treatment program. Their procedure requires speakers to nominate speaking intervals in which either type of speech will be used. Unfortunately, without independent measures of this variable(s), it is difficult to determine whether speakers can manipulate speech monitoring. But, more importantly, it is not clear how much, or what form of monitoring is desirable for normal speech behavior. Related to this is Webster's (1974) attempt to partially evaluate outcome from the Hollins program by asking listeners on follow-up questionnaires to indicate "how much attention must you pay to the task of speaking fluently?" This may help determine whether posttreatment effects oblige speakers to concentrate excessively on their "fluency." These preliminary efforts at measuring for monitoring of speech may have some problems, but, at present, no efforts have been made to measure the spontaneity that Bloodstein believes is necessary for normally fluent speech.

8. Treatment must remove not only stuttering, but also the sense of handicap and the person's self-concept as a stutterer.

This type of criterion is often presumed to present a special challenge to treatments that are mainly concerned with modifying or removing stuttering. It is assumed that a "sense of handicap," or a stutterer's "self-concept" are constructs that either retain the problem or are the essence of the problem. And, more significantly, it is assumed that their removal or alteration is necessary to the treatment's success. However, no data have ever shown that changes in stuttering do not also influence the "sense of handicap," or change the talker's concept of himself as a talker. That is not to suggest that patterns of behavior associated with stuttering will readily and immediately change when the disorder is modified. It would be rather surprising, for example, if embarrassing or constantly avoided circumstances were suddenly of no concern when stuttering ceases. Again, no data have shown that the persistence of such reactions is essentially abnormal or prevents normal fluency.

Surprisingly, Bloodstein (1981) partly justifies this criterion by referring to Andrews and Cutler's (1974) claim that the removal of stuttering in one situation was not sufficient to change stutterers' attitudes towards speaking. In fact, Andrew and Cutler's data actually show that when treatment was extended to other situations (in the course of a transfer procedure), the attitude scores showed concomitant and favorable changes. This aligns with findings from a subsequent investigation by Ulliana and Ingham (1984) on the attitude scale (S24) used in Andrews and Cutler's study which shows that the scale's scores are probably strongly influenced by the frequency of stuttering that occurs in situations referenced in the scale's items. In other words, it is highly likely that the "attitudinal factors" measured by the S24 are simply correlates of stuttering frequency. There is no reason to expect that a "sense of handicap," or "self-concept," might not also be related to actual stuttering frequency. In short, there is no evidence (to date) that such variables need particular attention within treatment in order to ensure therapy success.

9. The success of a program of therapy should not be inflated by ignoring dropouts.

Numerous examples of this problem exist in the stuttering treatment literature (Ingham, 1984). This is a problem in almost all areas of treatment research and, when excessive, prevents any meaningful conclusions from a study. The problem may well be much greater than is evident from studies in which large scale dropouts have been reported. For example, in single-subject studies it is very rarely indicated that the treated subjects were the *only* subjects on whom the procedure was tried. This information can be exceedingly important, as is demonstrated by numerous subjects who have dropped out of haloperidol treatment programs (Ingham, 1984). Their response probably reflects the less savory effects of this treatment, and serves to contraindicate haloperidol as a preferred treatment for stuttering (Guitar, 1984). Obviously the true clinical value of many treatments can only emerge when clinical researchers carefully ascertain the reasons for dropouts, and also report on nonresponders in the course of single-subject research.

10. The method must be shown to be effective in the hands of essentially any qualified clinician, including those without unusual status, prestige, or force of personality.

and

11. The method must continue to be successful when it is no longer new and the initial wave of enthusiasm over it has died away.

These are much related criteria that refer to the treatment's replicability and clinical viability. Actually, these criteria appear to have been met by many of the current therapy procedures, although most "replication" studies invariably highlight the contribution of additional treatment factors or therapy variations and are probably conducted by particularly enthusiastic clinicians. At the same time, an increasing number of treatment reports are now being written to reveal both the strengths and weaknesses of certain procedures, especially those using prolonged speech and its variants (Ingham, 1984). This is a vital shift in much stuttering therapy research and meets the spirit of Bloodstein's criterion. At the same time, many of the response contingent and prolonged speech treatment programs are continuing to produce benefits even now that the "initial wave of enthusiasm" has receded.

Bloodstein's (1981) criteria highlight most of the critical issues that need consideration in evaluating stuttering therapy. Some of the criteria seem questionable, most notably Criteria 1 and 8, but in general they are useful guides to stuttering therapy evaluation. Their limitation is that they are relatively nonspecific guides and provide insufficient information to help clinicians evaluate their own therapy endeavors. The purpose of clinical research is not only to design and evaluate treatments but also to improve therapy practice. So, in what follows, an attempt will be made to develop a set of guidelines for measuring treatment efficacy in therapy management. These guidelines will embrace most of Bloodstein's criteria and include a distillation of pertinent findings from recent clinical research.

TOWARDS A THERAPY EVALUATION SYSTEM

The purpose here is to develop a therapy evaluation system suitable for most stuttering therapy procedures. It is not posed as a "final solution" but draws on the current treatment literature to derive some necessary operations that should accompany therapy. Actually, any search for an all-purpose treatment evaluation design seems to have about as much chance of succeeding as the search for the Holy Grail. Indeed, the problem in such a search is to be able to recognize treatment success. For, if the object of stuttering therapy is to produce normally fluent speech, then that objective continues to be hindered by the absence of measures (or sets of measures) that can be used to describe normal fluency (Starkweather, 1980). But if clinicians are prepared to settle for an assessment strategy that shows when stuttering is changing as a function of treatment, and when some of the presumed relevant features of normal fluency are evident, then perhaps the search will not be fruitless.

One potential impediment to the search is the differing therapy formats among stuttering treatments. There are obvious differences between treatments concerned with directly modifying stuttering and those that treat stuttering by modifying other behaviors. That is not a major impediment, however, because all ultimately aim to modify stuttering, and so their efficacy can probably be related to various speech performance measures. More problematic is whether treatment is delivered intensively or intermittently. Because intensive treatment should produce improved speech more rapidly, the format will need sufficient flexibility to accommodate different expected rates of change. Thus within- and beyond-clinic assessments may need to be made relatively more frequently for intensive programs. Nevertheless, even this problem is surmountable provided the format's principal components and the guidelines for identifying therapy effects are suitable for both methods. Another difficulty might be the age of clients; there is some indication (Ingham, 1984) that children may be more responsive to certain treatments than adolescents or adults. It is possible that this difference might extend to rates of change, plus any criteria for determining clinically significant improvement. The same arguments could apply to differences in the intellectual level of clients, for there is also some indication that retardates respond more slowly to treatment (Ingham, 1984). The resolution of each of these difficulties is reasonably straightforward if the format is derived empirically. In other words, where data exist that demand exceptional formats, then such formats should be formulated.

Formulating the Evaluation System

The most significant lesson learned from the checkered history of stuttering therapy is that a useful treatment evaluation system should be designed so that it can embrace the known and anticipated variability of stuttering. It must be a system that is capable of demonstrating that therapy progress or outcome is not confounded by the known untreated variability of the subject's stuttering. Treatment evaluation formats that are suitable for this purpose are beginning to emerge from the time-series quasi-experimental designs (Hersen and Barlow, 1976) typically used in within-subject research. They are especially suitable because they not only identify variability, but also help deal with concerns such as accountability, decision making, and outcome evaluation. Furthermore, they are not only the most powerful designs available for determining sources of within-subject variability, but they are also the only ones that will enable the clinician to discern whether therapy is responsible for generalization.

The strength, or internal and external validity, of these designs in a therapy evaluation system depends on data collection within and beyond the therapy setting at clinically relevant intervals before, during, and after treatment. In short, the foundation of the recommended system is an integration of the now familiar multiple baseline and ABA designs. But the clinical viability of this system depends on finding some basis for determining clinically significant frequency, duration, and content of measurement within the system's design. The rationale for one such determination will now be outlined.

The Data Base, or What to Measure

There is probably little argument that an appropriate evaluation system requires access to audio-recorded speech within relevant speaking situations. Perhaps these recordings could be supplemented by video recordings to ensure that the visual aspects of stuttering (especially for severity measurement) are taken into account. In the absence of this facility, there is value in utilizing directly observed performance data.

Perhaps the minimal clinical data would be stuttering frequency counts and syllables (or words) spoken during talking time. They provide the bases for calculating percentages of syllables (or words) stuttered and syllables (or words) per minute—two of the most commonly used indices for recording the speech behavior of stutterers. These measures in turn assist clinicians in gauging changes in stuttering and the contribution that the amount and rate of speaking make to stuttering variability.

Stuttering Counts. The frequency of "moments of stuttering" may not fully depict the extent of disability caused by stuttering. However, this measure has certainly passed the test of time. The virtue of stuttering frequency counts is that they can be integrated with treatment via on-line measurement, while assessing the treatment's success (or otherwise) in removing the crux of the disorder. Most current therapies aim to remove all instances of stuttering, so it is becoming less important that those instances be described as more or less "severe" or as "part-word repetitions," etc. It also makes little sense now to confound stuttering counts with counts of normal disfluencies. There is increasing acceptance that clinicians (and certainly lay observers) are able to distinguish between disfluencies and stutterings (MacDonald and Martin, 1973).[3] This is an important point because there is no obvious advantage in a treatment that removes normal disfluencies but is less successful in removing stutterings. Conversely, a treatment that removes all disfluencies, normal and abnormal, may actually succeed in producing unusual fluency.

There are at least two dangers in relying on frequency counts of stuttering alone in order to evaluate treatment. The first relates to severity. Occasionally, a very low frequency of stuttering may contain exceptionally long moments of stuttering (Ingham, 1981). For this reason, there is good cause to record the duration or visible features of low frequency stuttering. The second reason concerns the role of word avoidance. This must be the least researched stuttering phenomenon, yet one of the best known features of the disorder—especially in adults. Perhaps the only way of measuring its presence is the subject's report and instructional tests for its influence. The latter may be ascertained by asking the subject to try to minimize stuttering for an interval, possibly by "avoiding stutterings" during spontaneous speech, and then comparing this interval with another in which the reverse instruction is given.

Speech Rate. The primary reason for measuring speech rate is that it is generally accepted that reduced speech rate may be sufficient to produce reduced stuttering. Of course, reduced speaking as such would have the same effect. Less publicized is the possibility that an abnormally fast speech rate may also reduce stuttering (Ingham, Martin, and Kuhl, 1974). However, there is no accepted method for measuring speech rate. One stumbling block is the relationship between existing rate measures and normally fluent speech rate. Speech rate measurement, as Starkweather (1980) has recently pointed out, needs to be much more complex than simple counts of words or syllables per minute. For what is a perceived as "fast" or "slow" turns out to be partially relative, but also dependent upon variables such as sound durations, pause durations, coarticulation, and rate of syllable production. Consequently, the currently used clinical measures of speech rate only approximate what is a perceived rate, or what might be a normal rate. In light of this, what options are available?

For some years the senior author and colleagues have used 170 to 210 syllables per minute as a target normal speech rate (Ingham, 1981). But this measure (allowing for its imperfections) is based on a relatively unusual speaking condition: a monologue that is not interrupted by the conversational exchanges typical of most speech behavior; plus it is the speech rate of young adults. Furthermore, these overall syllable-per-minute scores are neither as useful nor, probably, as valid as Perkins's (1975) measure of articulation rate which excludes pauses and occurrences of stuttering. However, in the absence of pertinent speech rate data, both measures probably provide different, but clinically useful, measures of rate during therapy (Costello, 1981; Costello and Ingham, 1984).

Another reflection of the need for research in this area is that there is little information on the relevant target speech rates that should pertain to the subject's age. There are some data from school children that indicate that the average syllable-per-minute rates in normal speech progressively increase throughout childhood. Kowal, O'Connell, and Sabin (1975) have shown that in kindergarten years this rate is about 50 per cent of adult rates and rises to near adult rates by around 12 years. At present, those data might provide the best guide for estimating the expected syllable-per-minute rates for different age groups at the end of treatment. Perhaps a better alternative, certainly one worthy of investigation, is the subject's natural speech rate during stutter-free intervals. Admittedly, these intervals (depending on their length) may be influenced by stuttering frequency, but they may also be more appropriate bases for determining the talker's "normally" fluent rate. Actually, the clinician's perceptual judgment of what is an acceptable and normal rate may ultimately translate into the most clinically suitable syllable-per-minute scores for the individual case— especially if speech normalcy or naturalness ultimately emerges as a reliable basis for determining this measure.

There are numerous reasons why speech rate and stuttering frequency measures are necessary, yet incomplete, for assessing speech performance in treatment. The most important is the imperfect connection between zero stuttering at "normal" speech rate and speech that is perceived as normally fluent (Ingham, 1981; Perkins, 1981). The need to improve this connection largely stems from the proliferation of treatments that procure "fluency" via unusual speech patterns, such as the variants of prolonged speech. Adams (1982), for example, has been particularly concerned about the need to gain much more information on the indices needed to identify normally fluent speech. Starkweather (1980) also explored these issues and concluded that fluent speech "is the quality of speech that includes rapid and easy, as well as smooth production" (p. 195). But, as yet, no known combination of measurement operations quantifies that speech quality.

Speech Quality. A number of approaches to the task of measuring speech quality have already been mentioned. These include ratings of naturalness, prosody, rate, and fluency, plus perceptual analyses of differences between speech samples from nonstutterers and treated stutterers. These measures may evaluate the results of treatment but, unfortunately, they cannot be readily integrated with the treatment process in the same fashion as stuttering counts and rate. However, one promising development, as was previously described, it is the use of on-line ratings of naturalness, provided it is possible to establish the reliability and validity of such ratings.

In general terms, therefore, measures that have maximum utility in a therapy context are those that yield dual-function data: (1) they provide bases for establishing within- and beyond-clinic treatment effects, and (2) they contribute to treatment operations (i.e., can be used on-line during treatment). Such dual function measures may not aid all therapies, but for most current therapies they should serve the first function. In passing, it is interesting to note the increasing recognition of the value of measures that do more than passively chart the subject's progress through therapy. Indeed, measures that permit decisions about the efficacy of therapy may have an integral role as treatment agents. It is this latter function that is being used lately to assist the transfer and maintenance of therapy effects (Ingham, 1980, 1982a).

Where to Collect Data

The crux of the system described herein is the establishment of multiple "standard" measures of the client's speech performance within and beyond the treatment setting. The conditions of such measures should be determined individually for each client so that they provide representative samples to tap the variability inherent in speaking performance within and beyond the clinic. These standard measures would, then, be administered regularly and repeatedly throughout the course of the clinician's (or clinical researcher's) clinical relationship with the client.

Within-Clinic Measures. It is well known (but not well documented) that stuttering may vary considerably across different speaking tasks and situations (Bloodstein, 1981; Guitar, 1975; Ingham and Packman, 1977; Resick et al., 1978; Ryan, 1974). A variety of within-clinic measures have been used rather arbitrarily in the literature, their usefulness being determined partly by the information they give regarding relevant parameters of the client's speech performance and, partly, by the convenience they offer to the clinician. What should be regarded as necessary? The most obvious contenders are conversational speech, monologues, and oral reading, because they are useful not only for assessment but are typically treatment activities as well. Oral reading is included mainly because of its utility in certain therapies; otherwise, it seems strange that so many stuttering assessment procedures recommend a task that is rarely performed in the natural environment (except occasionally in the school setting). Nevertheless, it does have the presumed advantage of controlling for avoidance. Clinician-client conversations and telephone conversations, both heavily laced with questions, are obviously good choices. The latter task is especially useful because of its suitability for beyond-clinic treatment and assessment as well. The ideal duration for each task is yet another "unknown," but in the context of demands on clinician time, perhaps each should be three minutes.

Beyond-Clinic Measures. The choice of the situations in which the subject's speech should be measured will be conditioned by the recordability of the situation as much as its validity. The recording process has been greatly assisted by the availability of exceedingly small, good quality microcassette recorders that should be within the resources of a clinic or a client. They can be worn comfortably and equipped with remote hand controls that simplify recording in most situations.

The choice of recordable assessment situations presents some complicated, but not unsolvable, difficulties. There are some logical choices: parents or spouse, peers, and significant others, and a reasonable cross-section of regularly occurring occasions where the client talks. The frequency and variety of talking situations occurring for individual stutterers could be derived with reasonable precision from logs kept by the client (or the client's parent) previous to enrollment in the treatment program (Darley and Spriestersbach, 1978). The number of beyond-clinic measures regularly obtained for each client will differ according to the breadth and frequency of a given client's talking occasions. The goal is that the clinician's (or experimenter's) beyond-clinic samples reflect the variability that would be found were it possible to have data on all of the client's speech throughout every day. (See Ingham and Packman, 1977, for an example of such continuous and complete measurement.) Typical beyond-clinic measures for children might contain standard samples of talking with the family during dinner, with a sibling during playtime, with the mother while riding in the car, and at school during "show and tell" and reading group. The typical adult client might provide recordings of speech from typical work situations, frequently occurring social situations, and conversations with his or her spouse at home.

The validity of the selected situations may be aided by two other considerations: use of the client's self-judged "difficult" (but recordable) situations, and the relative frequency with which these situations occur. These additional considerations should certainly be included within the decision base for choosing samples from the client's environment. A logical starting point for deciding the length each sample should be is that it reflect the client's typical talking time in similar settings. For example, if a child's speech with a parent occupies, say, 50 per cent of his or her estimated talking time, then recordings of similar talking should account for about 50 per cent of the beyond-clinic data collected for that client.

When to Collect Data

Reaching an agreeable decision about the frequency and duration of samples in a repeated measures assessment design involves at least three considerations: identifying variability, establishing that a treatment is "working," and managing data. However, taking account of these considerations in a generally acceptable therapy format is like putting together a jigsaw puzzle that has its pieces shaped by special interest groups whose members can never agree—arguably one common characteristic in this field. Nevertheless, there may be some parts of the puzzle that can be solved using compromise pieces.

Perhaps the first puzzle piece—identifying variability—should come from the ranks of clinical researchers. The difficulty is that these persons also offer little guidance on the minimum number of data points needed to reflect variability. For compromise purposes, therefore, perhaps the much referenced text by Hersen and Barlow (1976) should be a guide. They recommend at least three "data points" in any phase of an evaluation design employing data trend comparisons, although many of their text's examples use four or more data points for this purpose. Perhaps, therefore, the seemingly small number of four is an acceptable starting point. But does this translate into measuring relevant behavior for four consecutive days, once every four weeks, or perhaps, once every four months? This piece of the puzzle should probably come from two interest groups: practicing clinicians and the editors of journals reporting treatment studies, for it relates to the frequency with which treatment is offered, and the interval of time needed to convince peers that treatment efficacy has been established. The factors involved in constructing this piece will be deferred for the moment. The third, and most overlooked factor, is the sheer task of data collecting from audio recordings, and the subject's ability to obtain such recordings.

Determining a Treatment Effect

Once a suitable measurement schedule has been determined and introduced during the pretreatment period, it is continued throughout the instatement and transfer phases of the program. The next task is to find a suitable time frame that can be used to decide whether or not the therapy procedures are beneficial. This could lead to a veritable Pandora's box— comparing different therapies and their effects. Fortunately, the interior of the box is not as daunting as might be expected. We can at least take advantage of a body of therapy literature to gain some idea of the rate of change in target behaviors from successfully treated clients. Indeed, if that literature cannot be used for this purpose, then it has virtually no external validity (Birnbrauer, 1981). At the very least, it should show the expected rate of change in stuttering if a client responds to a particular treatment. For example, if the chosen treatment was one of the response contingent procedures, then perhaps a less dramatic decline in stuttering frequency should be expected when compared with rhythm or any of the numerous variants of prolonged speech. On the other hand, the relevant target behavior for these speech pattern techniques is usually eventual restoration of normal speech rate, thus extending the time needed ultimately to determine treatment responsiveness.

There is no reason to skirt the "treatment effect time" issue with generalities because much of the reviewed treatment literature—at least that which provides single-subject data—is able to be summarized for this purpose. Tables 8-1 and 8-2 provide summaries of the treatment studies that permit estimates of the treatment time required for stuttering or disfluencies (sometimes "dysfluencies") to decrease by at least 50 per cent relative to baserate. The term "successful outcome" is used in a very broad sense. It refers to those subjects who were reported, at the end of their treatment, to have reduced stuttering by at least 50 per cent without decreased speech rate (when these data are reported). A 50 per cent reduction in stutterings is certainly far from absolute treatment success, but, in the spirit of compromise, it is regarded as evidence that a substantial change in performance has been achieved by the treatment. The successfully treated subjects have been divided into children, those 12 years of age or younger (see Table 8-1), and adults (see Table 8-2). This is for no special reason, other than the recurring suggestion in the literature that children appear to respond more rapidly to some treatments than adults. Generally the tables confirm that children do respond a shade more rapidly to most treatment procedures, particularly the response contingent techniques. The

Table 8–1. This table summarizes the results of a survey of stuttering treatments involving children 12 years of age or younger. The survey was designed to identify studies in which it was possible to discern the treatment time needed for individual subjects to reduce stuttering or disfluencies by more than 50% relative to pretreatment performance. That point was established when the target behavior reached the 50% reduction level on two assessment occasions. In the case of "Gradual Increase in Length and Complexity of Utterance" (GILCU), the 50% reduction level was regarded as equivalent to half the time required to achieve the designated treatment target. For the speech pattern procedures, the 50% reduction level was regarded as equivalent to half the time required to complete the treatment's instatement phase.

Method	Procedure	Study	Hours Required for 50% Reduction in Target Behavior	Number of Subjects/ Age Range
Response Contingent	GILCU	Costello (1980)	15.50	1/11
		Johnson, Coleman, and Rasmussen (1978)	10.50	1/6
		Ryan (1974)	3.30–30.05	6/7–9
		Mowrer (1975)	5.00	1/10
	Positive Reinforcement	Peters (1977)	0.60	2/8
		Shaw and Shrum (1972)	0.67	3/9–10
	Combined Punishment and Reinforcement	Ryan (1974)	1.00–6.00	2/9

Table 8-1 (continued)

Punishment	Martin and Berndt (1970)	0.67	1/12
	Martin, Kuhl, and Haroldson (1972)	1.33–2.00	2/3–4
	McDermott (1971)	1.20	1/9
	Reed and Godden (1977)	1.33–1.67	2/3–5
Masking Continuous	MacCulloch, Eaton, and Long (1970)	6.00	4/11.9
Speech Pattern Rhythmic Stimulation	Herscovitch and Le Bow (1973)	2.00	2/12
MCSR	Brady (1971)	4.00	1/12
DAF/ Prolonged Speech	Ryan (1971)	2.00	1/8
	Ryan (1974)	5.65–20.25	2/8–12
	Turnbaugh and Guitar (1981)	4.50	1/12
Speech Pattern Regulated Breathing	Hee and Holmes (1976)	1.50	1/10
Shadowing	Ottoni (1974)	1.00	1/9
Traditional Programmed	Ryan (1974)	2.30	1/10

Table 8-2. Table incorporates the same information as Table 8-1 but for subjects older than 12 years

Method	Procedure	Study	Hours Required for 50% Reduction in Target Behavior	Number of Subjects/ Age Range
Response Contingent	GILCU	Mowrer (1975)	5.00–9.75	2/23,31
		Ryan (1974)	5.25–19.30	3/16–35
	Punishment	Costello (1975)	1.83	1/18
		Ryan (1974)	3.05–5.15	2/15,20
	Self-management	James (1981)	23.00	1/18
		La Croix (1973)	1.00	2/?
Anxiety Reduction	Reciprocal Inhibition	Boudreau and Jeffrey (1973)	12.00	4/16–22
Speech Pattern	Rhythmic Stimulation	Brady (1971)	5.00–31.00	17/14–53

Table 8–2 (continued)

Prolonged Speech	Andrews (1973)	5.00	1/?
	Boberg and Fong (1980)	15.00	1/19
DAF/ Prolonged Speech	Goldiamond (1965)	3.08	2/40,?
	Ingham and Andrews (1973)	1.63–4.60	11/18–56
	Ryan (1974)	1.00–88.60	23/14–45
	Webster (1970)	5.00–20.00	8/15–47
Biofeeback EMG	Guitar (1975)	2.67	1/32
Traditional Programmed	Ryan (1974)	1.45–12.05	9/14–43

rate of response to the GILCU and speech pattern techniques are more difficult to translate since there is no clear indication of the time taken to reach 50 per cent improvement. For this reason, half the treatment time, or talking time, required to reach the final target behavior was judged equivalent to 50 per cent improvement. This is probably the main reason why these treatments appear to take longer to reach the "treatment effect" criterion.

Resolving the Treatment Design Puzzle

The next task is to translate the preceding information into solution pieces for the treatment design puzzle. The first issue must be the frequency with which baseline and subsequent measures during and after treatment should be made. Andrews and Harvey (1981) have gathered data that they suggest show that pretreatment speech measures from adult stutters do not show improvement over a 6-week nontreatment period. Thus, the most conservative treatment design might incorporate up to 6 weeks of weekly recordings of the subject's speech within and beyond the clinic prior to the initiation of treatment. The least conservative, though possibly the most practical, approach might utilize the four-data-point principle, with a minimum of, say, once weekly recordings of all selected within- and beyond-clinic speech samples. This would seem to provide adequate sampling of the existing variability in the client's stuttering across settings and time.

Clinicians should be aware that this recommended 4-week baserate data collection interval is not necessarily a period of clinical inactivity. It is during this period that the clinician might train the client's spouse or parents not only to collect appropriate beyond-clinic recordings but also to score these recordings reliably. Also, in some instances the authors have found that the baserate recording procedure, per se, appears to have produced "treatment effects," thus influencing subsequent intervention decisions. Finally, the baserate period can be used to organize the format of treatment procedures. The methods for choosing these procedures are considered in more detail by Costello and Ingham (1984).

Tables 8–1 and 8–2 suggest that the treatment phase for almost all current data-based treatments should not exceed about 12 treatment hours for children or 23 hours of treatment for adults, before a decision is made as to whether the chosen treatment should be continued or changed. Actually, quite discernible trends in relevant data should be expected by the fifth hour if some treatments are likely to be beneficial. Of course, this does not mean the treatment will be ultimately successful, since it is likely that many treatment failures showed evidence of responsiveness within the suggested time frames. On the other hand, relatively few successful treatments demonstrated responsiveness over longer intervals.

If treatment is progressing appropriately, at some point within-clinic and beyond-clinic data will begin to converge until speech performance under all conditions has reached criterion. At this point, the clinician will need to make some decision about the number of data collection occasions that are needed to verify that change and thus indicate the appropriateness of termination of the establishment-transfer phase of treatment. The simple fact is that there are almost no data that can be used to address this issue. Perhaps the sole exception occurs in a single-subject study by Ingham and Packman (1977). Obviously, more data are needed to address this issue, one research area in which group data would be useful. In the absence of such data, the clinician might be best advised to rely on the data collection intervals used thus far throughout baseline and treatment. These will provide at least one source for determining whether clinically significant changes have resulted from treatment. Perhaps, therefore, the client's performance pattern over 4 beyond- and within-clinic data collection points, while treatment has ceased, might be one rational basis for deciding whether maintenance procedures should be introduced to the therapy process. However, there are more complex issues associated with assessing treatment outcome that will be discussed later.

Dismantling Therapy

It may well be that a number of treatments are tried before a therapy strategy is found that will achieve within- and beyond-clinic treatment gains. These will be strategies that establish and transfer treatment gains. It is, therefore, necessary for the assessment process to incorporate strategies that will indicate when the initial phase of treatment (i.e., establishment and, if necessary, transfer) should be replaced by maintenance strategies.

There is general agreement that active maintenance strategies are necessary components of the therapy process, although that is often difficult to believe considering the slight amount of research they have attracted. There are some very limited data available that demonstrate the efficacy of some maintenance techniques (Boberg, 1981; Boberg, Howie, and Woods, 1977; Ingham, 1980, 1981, 1982a), though they give no guidance on how to choose assessment procedures for this phase. To some extent, that task has been eased by some useful data that suggest that when beyond-clinic generalization occurs in the treatment of preschool children, then unassisted maintenance will follow (Ingham, 1984; Prins and Ingham, 1983). But the evidence is certainly not so persuasive in the case of older children.

As mentioned earlier, repeated beyond- and within-clinic assessments at the end of treatment should continue over at least four data collection points. This should provide a reasonable basis for estimating the initial stability of these gains. However, the dismantling of the therapy process may also blend with treatment and assessment procedures. One internally valid method of establishing when treatment should be withdrawn is to use a period when the beyond- or within-clinic data collection scores (i.e., nontreatment scores) and therapy-controlled measures of speech performance begin to merge. Martin, Kuhl, and Haroldson (1972) demonstrated the prospects of this strategy when they compared treatment and nontreatment setting performance of two preschool stutterers treated by contingency arrangements. Costello (1975) used this strategy during therapy sessions by comparing nontreatment and treatment intervals over contingency-managed therapy sessions.

A strategy used by the senior author in recent years (Ingham, 1980, 1981, 1982a) involves systematic withdrawal of regular assessment sessions contingent upon sustained performance, plus comparisons with intermittent covert assessments. This is also an example of how beyond-clinic (or within-clinic) assessments can serve dual functions; that is, they decrease the contact frequency with the client but remain a useful source of speech control.

The above-mentioned method for continuing maintenance and evaluation illustrates how maintenance and outcome evaluation strategies may be gradually integrated. In this procedure the subject is required to return to the clinic initially for two once-weekly assessments, and if the target behavior (0 per cent syllables stuttered at between 170 and 210 SPM) is maintained in all within- and beyond-clinic assessments, then the subject "earns" a 2-week rest from assessments. If these 2 week apart assessments achieve the target behavior, then the subject earns a 4-week rest from assessments. This systematic and performance-contingent withdrawal of assessment continues until two 32 week apart assessments are passed successfully. If the subject fails on any assessment (that is, has one stuttering or departs from the target speech rate on any task), then the weekly assessments are reinstated. Recently this procedure was successfully used in conjunction with a self-management technique (specifically, self-evaluation training) in order to shift the responsibility for conducting this performance-contingent assessment strategy to the subject (Ingham, 1982a). These procedures have been mainly used with adults, but they have also been useful with older children (Ingham, 1980). Of most relevance here is the fact that the data from these studies have been supplemented by nonperformance-contingent assessments made in beyond-clinic conditions, thereby establishing the point when the data from the nontreatment-related assessments blend with those from the treatment-related assessments. They have also been supplemented by a wide variety of covert assessments that have shown, in some cases, that data gained from overt and covert assessments differ markedly. Generally, these concurrent assessments indicate that the maintenance strategy may be phased out well before the 32 week apart assessment point.

Covert Assessment. Undoubtedly, covert assessment procedures are among the most contentious assessment techniques used in stuttering therapy. Some recent group studies (Howie, Woods, and Andrews, 1982; Andrews and Craig, 1982) have questioned their worth by finding that covert and overt group data are not significantly different 6 months or more after treatment. But studies on individuals (Ingham, 1980, 1982a) have shown that the data from both sources may be quite different well after the initial phase of treatment has ceased. In consequence, covert assessments certainly have the potential of providing the most clinically valid treatment assessment data, particularly when used in conjunction with relevant overt assessment data. Their claim to validity, however, is only as strong as their claim to be unobtrusive—and these claims are often difficult to defend. There are various types of covert and perhaps not-so-covert assessment techniques that might be relatively free of the reactive features of overt assessment, features that many clinicians suspect produce "artificial" posttreatment data. Perhaps the most useful is the "unplanned telephone call," made, ideally, by a person not associated with the treatment. Other relevant information may be obtained from the subject's associates, and can then be validated by carefully arranged recordings. Admittedly, this all sounds uncomfortably unethical, but it need not be. In the case of older children, adolescents, and adults, it is unlikely that the assessment's validity will be threatened if, before treatment, the client agrees that such assessments will only be used to test the treatment's worth. The authors have often used this procedure over the past decade, and have yet to meet one client who found it to be unacceptable. More importantly, it has often provided an immensely useful clinical service. For instance, if repeated unobtrusive assessments yield evidence of poorer performance compared to other, more directly obtained measures, then the consequent trend of performance scores can be used to determine the merit of continuing an extraclinic treatment procedure. When the extraclinic covert data fail to show improvement, then it may be necessary to integrate such data with treatment. For example, in the current applications of the above-described maintenance schedule, clinicians intermittently telephone subjects. If the clinician detects stuttering, then, regardless of whether the subject "passed" the previous assessment, the subject automatically fails that assessment and returns to the initial step in the maintenance schedule.

How should covert assessments be organized within an assessment schedule? Like all other assessment decisions, the decision to use covert assessment should be guided, where possible, by treatment and evaluation considerations. However, the difficulty with this form of assessment is that its "cover" is vulnerable if it is used too frequently. This type of assessment probably carries adequate treatment and assessment value if it occurs on at least four occasions during the transfer phase and on another four occasions during the immediate posttreatment assessment phase. This allows the clinician to decide whether the subject's assessed speech performance is reflected in less stimulus-bound conditions. Probably the most practical procedure for the purpose is an unannounced telephone conversation with a person unconnected with the treatment. It is up to the clinician to decide how the data should be obtained, but there is no reason why it cannot be assessed on-line by a trained clinician. The frequency with which covert assessments should be made during the maintenance phase depends largely on the duration of that phase. Of course, in turn, this raises the issue of time spans for posttreatment assessments, the final phase of this suggested format.

Followup Assessment

To date, our literature has little information that could be used to justify the use of certain prescribed followup intervals or followup assessments. The typical recommendations are that posttreatment assessments should occur at intervals ranging from a few weeks to 5 years (Silverman, 1981). What this reflects is yet another area of confusion, this time about the function of posttreatment evaluation. The primary purpose of the followup evaluation is surely to establish whether the client is unimproved, improved, or free of his or her problem after a period in which variables likely to influence the problem have had every opportunity to occur. The fact that a subject shows improvement, or otherwise, at followup may have very little to do with treatment. Quite clearly, the longer the interval between cessation of treatment and followup evaluation, the more likely it is that this interval will be filled with variables of far more relevance to current performance than the original treatment. Unfortunately, there is also little information available on the nature of these variables, but there are some logical contenders: practice regimes, "significant others," self-control of speech performance, and even additional treatment are good prospects for consideration.

At best, it would appear that followup evaluation may give the clinician and client knowledge about the current state of the disorder and some useful hypotheses about the durability of the treatment's effects. For this reason, perhaps the most practical guideline for followup evaluation is to schedule intermittent assessments over the following year. This will probably accommodate a clinic's annual time-tabling arrangements, and is consistent with the intervals used in many clinical studies.

The frequency of followup assessments presents another imponderable. Perhaps the logical solution is to use the "four-data-point" principle from the previously mentioned therapy assessment format. This means that followup assessments should occur at 3-month intervals. And in order to determine the validity of this trend, perhaps these assessments should be interspersed with another four covert assessments.

The content of these posttreatment assessments deserves additional comment. The logical contenders are the within- and beyond-clinic assessments used over the initial therapy phases. Perhaps the most practical option for covert assessment is a 3- to 5-minute surprise telephone call involving a question-answer conversation with a stranger. But at least two other assessments may be important: some form of assessment of the subject's speech quality (discussed above) and a questionnaire similar to those devised by Webster (1974) and Perkins (1981). The main value of Webster's questionnaire, for instance, is that it solicits the subject's judgment on the extent of attentiveness to self-monitoring required to continue to speak fluently. At present, no other means are available for determining the extent to which therapy gains are sustained at the cost of unusual levels of attention to speaking. Once again, there are no available norms for this part of Webster's questionnaire, but it might be expected that over the followup period there should be some evidence that the subject's level of attention to his speech declines in concert with sustained improvements. That would seem to be one final clinically valid indication of treatment success.

CONCLUSIONS

Let us now try to put together all the pieces of our therapy assessment puzzle. It begins when we have established the subject's suitability for therapy. This is followed by a baserate period containing repeated within-

and and beyond-clinic recorded assessments. There should be at least four once-weekly within- and beyond-clinic assessments over the baserate period which would, therefore, extend for four weeks. These assessments continue at this frequency during the establishment and transfer phases of therapy. When data from all within- and beyond-clinic measures show criterion performance for four consecutive assessments, formal treatment could be terminated. Thus, at the end of the establishment or transfer phase, beyond- and within-clinic assessments should continue for the same duration as the baserate in order to establish performance stability, or otherwise. The subsequent maintenance phase may include decreasingly frequent assessments that might also be tied to the treatment process. The pattern of maintenance assessments should continue until they occur at 3-month intervals. At this point, they should fade into followup assessments made at 3-month intervals over a year.

The overt within- and beyond-clinic assessment procedure utilized throughout the preceding format should be supplemented by at least four unobtrusive or covert assessments made during both the treatment and transfer phases, plus another four assessments during the immediate posttreatment phase. In addition, perhaps covert assessments (of one form or another) should be made at regular intervals over the maintenance and followup periods. The content of the overt assessments should include representative speech samples from the client's natural environment, plus oral readings, monologues, and telephone conversations within the clinic.

The minimum data used in assessments should be syllables per minute or articulation rate, and percentage of syllables (or words) stuttered. These data should be supplemented by ratings of speech quality, especially during the final part of the treatment phase. The posttreatment phase of therapy might also include a questionnaire that solicits the subject's estimate of the extent to which it is necessary to "control" speech performance.

We hope that this suggested therapy management system will be given serious consideration as one means of shifting stuttering therapy towards a reasonably common pattern of assessment. This might help achieve a clearer understanding of the therapy process—an understanding that will be of immense benefit to all concerned with this disorder. There is an almost desperate need for a data base from field clinicians on the outcome of current stuttering therapy procedures. If clinicians could be encouraged to gather and report data within the suggested system, then the profession should be considerably advanced in solving that need, for only clinicians can show the strengths and weaknesses of these treatments in the field, rather than in the research laboratory. At the same time, the use of this system would go some distance towards meeting Bloodstein's (1981) therapy evaluation criteria. Finally, it should be mentioned that the suggested therapy management system has already been used successfully in clinical conditions. Ingham and Onslow (1983) have prepared a Stuttering Treatment Evaluation Manual which incorporates guidelines on the use of the previously described procedures. There is every indication from the trial use of this manual with various clinicians in diverse settings that the procedures can be easily implemented.

[1]The content of this chapter takes as a starting point some ideas about stuttering treatment outcome evaluation that were first presented in Ingham (1982b) and further developed in Ingham (1984).

[2]The interested reader is urged to read Bloodstein's justification for each criterion.

[3]Less decisive findings have been reported by Curlee (1981).

REFERENCES

Adams, M. R. (1982). Fluency, nonfluency, and stuttering in children. *Journal of Fluency Disorders, 7,* 171–185.

Andrews, G. (1973). Stuttering therapy: How simple can an effective treatment programme become? *Australian Journal of Human Communication Disorders, 1,* 44–46.

Andrews, G., and Craig, A. (1982). Stuttering: Overt and covert measurement of the speech of treated subjects. *Journal of Speech and Hearing Disorders, 47,* 96–99.

Andrews, G., and Cutler, J. (1974). Stuttering therapy: The relation between changes in symptom level and attitudes. *Journal of Speech and Hearing Disorders, 39,* 312–319.

Andrews, G., Guitar, B., and Howie, P. (1980). Meta-analysis of the effects of stuttering treatment. *Journal of Speech and Hearing Disorders, 45,* 287–307.

Andrews, G., and Harvey, R. (1981). Regression to the mean in pretreatment measures of stuttering. *Journal of Speech and Hearing Disorders, 46,* 204–207.

Andrews, G., and Ingham, R. (1972). An approach to the evaluation of stuttering therapy. *Journal of Speech and Hearing Research, 15,* 296–302.

Birnbrauer, J. S. (1981). External validity and experimental investigation of individual behavior. *Analysis and Intervention in Developmental Disabilities, 1,* 117–132.

Bloodstein, O. (1981). *A handbook on stuttering* (3rd ed.). Chicago: National Easter Seal Society.

Boberg, E. (1981). *Maintenance of fluency.* New York: Elsevier.

Boberg, E., and Fong, L. (1980). Therapy program for young retarded stutterers. *Human Communication, 2,* 95–102.

Boberg, E., Howie, P., and Woods, C. L. (1979). Maintenance of fluency: A review. *Journal of Fluency Disorders, 4,* 93-116.

Boudreau, L. A., and Jeffrey, C. J. (1973). Stuttering treated by desensitization. *Journal of Behavior Therapy and Experimental Psychiatry, 4,* 209-212.

Brady, J. P. (1971). Metronome-conditioned speech retraining for stuttering. *Behavior Therapy, 2,* 129-150.

Costello, J. M. (1975). The establishment of fluency with time-out procedures: Three case studies. *Journal of Speech and Hearing Disorders, 40,* 216-231.

Costello, J. M. (1979). Clinicians and researchers: A necessary dichotomy? *Journal of the National Student Speech and Hearing Association, 7,* 6-26.

Costello, J. M. (1980). Operant conditioning and the treatment of stuttering. In W. H. Perkins (Ed.), *Strategies in stuttering therapy. Seminars in Speech, Language and Hearing, 1,* New York: Decker.

Costello, J. M. (1981). Pretreatment assessment of stuttering in young children. *Communicative Disorders: An Audio Journal for Continuing Education.* New York: Grune and Stratton.

Costello, J. M. (1982). Techniques of therapy based on operant theory. In W. H. Perkins (Ed.), *Current therapy of communication disorders.* New York: Thieme-Stratton.

Costello, J. M., and Ingham, R. J. (1984). Assessment strategies for child and adult stutterers. In W. Perkins and R. Curlee (Eds.), *Nature and treatment of stuttering: New directions.* San Diego: College-Hill Press.

Curlee, R. F. (1981). Observer agreement on disfluency and stuttering. *Journal of Speech and Hearing Research, 24,* 595-600.

Darley, F. L., and Spriestersbach, D. C. (1978). *Diagnostic methods in speech pathology.* New York: Harper and Row.

Eysenck, H. J. (1978). An exercise in mega-silliness. *American Psychologist, 33,* 517.

Goldiamond, I. (1965). Stuttering and fluency as manipulatable operant response classes. In L. Krasner and L. P. Ullmann (Eds.), *Research in behavior modification.* New York: Holt, Rinehart, and Winston.

Gregory, H. H. (Ed.) (1978). *Controversies about stuttering therapy.* Baltimore: University Park Press.

Guitar, B. (1975). Reduction of stuttering frequency using analog electromyographic feedback. *Journal of Speech and Hearing Research, 18,* 672-685.

Guitar, B. E. (1979). A response to Ingham's critique. *Journal of Speech and Hearing Disorders, 44,* 400-403.

Guitar, B. E. (1981). A correction to "A response to Ingham's critique." *Journal of Speech and Hearing Disorders, 46,* 440.

Guitar, B. E. (1984). The indirect treatment of stuttering. In J. M. Costello, *Speech disorders in children.* San Diego, College-Hill Press.

Guitar, B., and Bass, C. (1978). Stuttering therapy: The relationship between attitude change and long term outcome. *Journal of Speech and Hearing Disorders, 43,* 392-400.

Hanna, R., and Owen, N. (1977). Facilitating transfer and maintenance of fluency in stuttering therapy. *Journal of Speech and Hearing Disorders, 42,* 65-76.

Hawkins, R. P., and Dotson, V. A. (1975). Reliability scores that delude: An Alice in Wonderland trip through the misleading characteristics of interobserver agreement scores in interval recording. In E. Ramp and G. Semb (Eds.), *Behavior analysis: Areas of research and application.* Englewood Cliffs, NJ: Prentice-Hall.

Hee, J. C., and Holmes, P. A. (1976) Elimination of stuttering by a regulated breathing approach. *Journal of Communication Pathology, 8,* 40-44.

Herscovitch, A., and LeBow, M. D. (1973). Imaginal pacing in the treatment of stuttering. *Journal of Behavior Therapy and Experimental Psychiatry, 4,* 357-360.

Hersen, M., and Barlow, D. H. (1976). *Single-case experimental designs.* New York: Pergamon.

Howie, P. M., Woods, C. L., and Andrews, G. (1982). Relationship between covert and overt speech measures immediately before and immediately after stuttering treatment. *Journal of Speech and Hearing Disorders, 47,* 419–422.

Ingham, R. J. (1979). Comment on "Stuttering therapy: The relation between attitude change and long-term outcome." *Journal of Speech and Hearing Disorders, 44,* 397–400.

Ingham, R. J. (1980). Modification of maintenance and generalization in stuttering treatment. *Journal of Speech and Hearing Research, 23,* 732–745.

Ingham, R. J. (1981). Evaluation and maintenance in stuttering treatment: A search for ecstasy with nothing but agony. In E. Boberg (Ed.), *Maintenance of fluency.* New York: Elsevier.

Ingham, R. J. (1982a). The effects of self-evaluation training on maintenance and generalization during stuttering treatment. *Journal of Speech and Hearing Disorders, 47,* 271–280.

Ingham, R. J. (1982b). *Towards a therapy assessment procedure for treating stuttering in children.* Paper presented at the Conference on Evaluation of Disfluency, Prevention of Stuttering, and Management of Fluency Problems in Children. Northwestern University, Evanston, IL.

Ingham, R. J. (1984). *Stuttering and behavior therapy: Current status and experimental foundations.* San Diego: College-Hill Press.

Ingham, R. J., and Andrews, G. (1973). An analysis of a token economy in stuttering therapy. *Journal of Applied Behavior Analysis, 6,* 219–229.

Ingham, R. J., Martin, R. R., and Kuhl, P. (1974). Modification and control of rate of speaking by stutterers. *Journal of Speech and Hearing Research, 17,* 489–496.

Ingham, R. J., and Onslow, M. (1983). *Stuttering treatment evaluation manual.* Sydney: Cumberland College of Health Sciences.

Ingham, R. J., and Packman, A. (1977). Treatment and generalization effects in an experimental treatment for a stutterer using contingency management and speech rate control. *Journal of Speech and Hearing Disorders, 42,* 394–407.

Ingham, R. J., and Packman, A. (1978). Perceptual assessment of normalcy of speech following stuttering therapy. *Journal of Speech and Hearing Research, 21,* 63–73.

James, J. E. (1981). Behavioral self-control of stuttering using time-out from speaking. *Journal of Applied Behavior Analysis, 14,* 25–37.

Johnson, G. F., Coleman, K., and Rasmussen, K. (1978). Multidays: Multidimensional approach for the young stutterer. *Language, Speech, and Hearing Services in Schools, 9,* 129–132.

Jones, R. J., and Azrin, N. H. (1969). Behavioral engineering: Stuttering as a function of stimulus duration during speech synchronization. *Journal of Applied Behavior Analysis, 2,* 223–229.

Kiesler, D. J. (1966). Some myths of psychotherapy research and the search for a paradigm. *Psychological Bulletin, 65,* 110–136.

Kowal, S., O'Connell, D. C., and Sabin, E. F. (1975). Development of temporal patterning and vocal hesitations in spontaneous narratives. *Journal of Psycholinguistic Research, 4,* 195–207.

LaCroix, Z. E. (1973). Management of disfluent speech through self-recording procedures. *Journal of Speech and Hearing Disorders, 38,* 272–274.

MacCulloch, M. J., Eaton, R., and Long E. (1970). The long term effect of auditory masking on young stutterers. *British Journal of Disorders of Communication, 5,* 165–173.

MacDonald, J. D., and Martin, R. R. (1973). Stuttering and disfluency as two reliable and unambiguous response classes. *Journal of Speech and Hearing Research, 16,* 691–699.

Martin, R. R. (1981). Appercus. In E. Boberg (Ed.), *Maintenance of fluency.* New York: Elsevier.

Martin, R. R., and Berndt, L. A. (1970). The effects of time-out on stuttering in a 12 year old boy. *Exceptional Children, 36,* 303–304.

Martin, R. R., and Haroldson, S. K. (1969). The effects of two treatment procedures on stuttering. *Journal of Communication Disorders, 2,* 115–125.

Martin, R. R., Haroldson, S. K., and Triden, K. A. (1984). Stuttering and speech naturalness. *Journal of Speech and Hearing Disorders, 49,* 53–58.

Martin, R. R., Kuhl, P., and Haroldson, S. K. (1972). An experimental treatment with two preschool stuttering children. *Journal of Speech and Hearing Research, 15,* 743–752.

McDermott, L. D. (1971). Clinical management of stuttering behavior: A case study. *Feedback, 1,* 6–7.

McReynolds, L. V., and Kearns, K. P. (1983). *Single-subject experimental designs in communicative disorders.* Baltimore: University Park Press.

Metz, D. E., Onufrak, J. A., and Ogburn, R. S. (1979). An acoustical analysis of stutterer's speech prior to and at the termination of therapy. *Journal of Fluency Disorders, 4,* 249–254.

Mowrer, D. (1975). An instructional program to increase fluent speech of stutterers. *Journal of Fluency Disorders 1,* 25–35.

Ottoni, T. M. (1974). Uso de la tecnica delineamento del habla para cambiar la conducta verbal. *Revista Interamericana de Psicologia, 8,* 3–4.

Perkins, W. H. (1975). Articulatory rate in the evaluation of stuttering treatments. *Journal of Speech and Hearing Disorders, 40,* 277–278.

Perkins, W. H. (1981). Measurement and maintenance of fluency. In E. Boberg (Ed.), *Maintenance of fluency.* New York: Elsevier.

Perkins, W. H., Rudas, J., Johnson, L., Michael, W. B., and Curlee, R. F. (1974). Replacement of stuttering with normal speech: III. Clinical effectiveness. *Journal of Speech and Hearing Disorders, 39,* 416–428.

Peters, A. D. (1977). The effect of positive reinforcement on fluency: Two case studies. *Language, Speech, and Hearing Services in Schools, 8,* 15–22.

Prins, D., and Ingham, R. J. (1983). *Treatment of stuttering in early childhood: Methods and issues.* San Diego: College-Hill Press.

Reed, C. G., and Godden, A. L. (1977). An experimental treatment using verbal punishment with two preschool stutterers. *Journal of Fluency Disorders, 2,* 225–233.

Resick, P. A., Wendiggensen, P., Ames, S., and Meyer, V. (1978). Systematic slowed speech: A new treatment for stuttering. *Behaviour Research and Therapy, 16,* 161–167.

Runyan, C. M., and Adams, M. R. (1978). Perceptual study of the speech of "successfully therapeutized" stutterers. *Journal of Fluency Disorders, 3,* 25–39.

Runyan, C. M., and Adams, M. R. (1979). Unsophisticated judges' perceptual evaluations of the speech of "successfully treated" stutterers. *Journal of Fluency Disorders, 4,* 29–38.

Ryan, B. P. (1971). Operant procedures applied to stuttering therapy for children. *Journal of Speech and Hearing Disorders, 36,* 264–280.

Ryan, B. P. (1974). *Programmed therapy for stuttering in children and adults.* Springfield, IL: Charles C Thomas.

Shames, G. H. (1981). Relapse in stuttering. In E. Boberg (Ed.), *Maintenance of fluency.* New York: Elsevier.

Shames, G. H., and Florance, C. L. (1980). *Stutter-free speech: A goal for therapy.* Columbus, OH: Charles E. Merrill.

Shaw, C. K., and Shrum, W. F. (1972). The effects of response-contingent reward on the connected speech of children who stutter. *Journal of Speech and Hearing Disorders, 37,* 75–88.

Sheehan, J. G. (1980). Problems in the evaluation of progress and outcome. *Seminars in Speech, Language, and Hearing, 1,* New York: Decker.

Silverman, F. H. (1981). Relapse following stuttering therapy. In N. J. Lass (Ed.), *Speech and language: Advances in basic research and practice* (Vol. 5). New York: Academic Press.

Smith, L. M., and Glass, G. (1977). Meta-analysis of psychotherapy outcome studies. *American Psychologist, 32,* 752-760.

Starkweather, C. W. (1980). Speech fluency and its development in normal children. In N.J. Lass (Ed.), *Speech and language: Advances in basic research and practice* (Vol. 4). New York: Academic Press.

Stokes, T. F., and Baer, D. M. (1977). An implicit technology of generalization. *Journal of Applied Behavior Analysis, 10,* 349-367.

Turnbaugh, K. R., and Guitar, B. E. (1981). Short-term intensive stuttering treatment in a public school setting. *Language, Speech, and Hearing Services in Schools, 12,* 107-114.

Ulliana, L., and Ingham, R. J. (1984). Behavioral and nonbehavioral variables in the measurement of stutterers' communication attitudes. *Journal of Speech and Hearing Disorders, 49,* 83-93.

Webster, R. L. (1970). Stuttering: A way to eliminate it and a way to explain it. In R. Ulrich, T. Stachnik, and J. Mabry (Eds.), *Control of human behavior* (Vol. 2). Glenview, IL: Scott Foresman.

Webster, R. L. (1974). *The Precision Fluency Shaping Program: Speech reconstruction for stutterers.* Roanoke, VA: Hollins Communication Research Institute.

Author Index

A

Abbs, J., 6, 7, 29, 30, 32, 36, 39, 41, 42, 44, 45, 46, 47, 49, 50
Adams, M. R., 159, 170, 179, 196, 203
Ahmed, M., 99
Aldes, M., 97
Alexander, R. M., 22
Ames, S., 193, 204
Aminoff, M., 87, 88
Andrews, A., 85
Andrews, G., 45, 47, 163, 164, 167, 172, 173, 174, 177, 178, 181, 190, 191, 192, 195, 198, 211, 212, 215
Ansberry, M., 157
Appenteng, K., 47
Armour, R., 12
Aronson, A., 3, 5, 6, 42, 44, 44, 87, 88, 128
Askenfelt, A., 86
Austin, D., 84
Azrin, N. H., 167, 168, 177, 178, 182, 196

B

Bacon, M., 84, 88
Baer, D. M., 181, 194
Baer, T., 85
Baird, C., 12
Baird, J., 12
Baken, R. J., 47, 89, 92, 95, 98
Baker, S. H., 118
Bankson, N. W., 74
Bannister, R., 86
Barlow, D. H., 190, 195, 201, 206
Barlow, S. M., 7, 36, 39, 42, 49
Barnes, H. E., 159
Barrington, C. C., 160
Barton, R., 100
Bashir, A., 12, 13
Bass, C., 162, 194
Bassich, C., 6, 85, 88
Battmer, R., 79
Batza, E., 100

Beck, M. A., 130, 138
Beckett, R. L., 137, 138, 139
Bell, J., 176
Bennett, M. H., 51
Benton, L. A., 22, 23
Berci, G., 85, 99
Berman, P. A., 159
Berndt, L. A., 170
Bernstein, N., 33
Bernthal, J. E., 74
Berry, W., 5
Beste, L. R., 130
Beukelman, D., 12
Beumer, J., 11, 12
Biller, H., 100
Birkmayer, W., 8
Birnbrauer, J. S., 207
Bjarkman, P. C., 70
Blom, E. D., 115, 118, 120, 121, 122, 123
Blonsky, E., 7, 8, 88
Blood, G., 96
Bloodstein, O., 157, 161, 164, 167, 190, 194, 198, 199, 204, 218
Blumstein, S., 6
Boberg, E., 194, 211, 213
Bocchino, J., 87
Boone, D., 6, 87, 128, 130, 135, 145, 146
Boothroyd, A., 92
Boshes, B., 88
Boudreau, L. A., 160, 177, 210
Bowers, M., 89
Bowman, J. P., 47
Brady, J. P., 159, 209, 210
Bralley, R., 95
Bratzlavsky, M., 47, 51
Brindle, B., 84
Broad, C., 89
Brodeur, 10
Brodnitz, F. S., 10, 11, 87, 93, 96, 127, 130
Brooks, V. B., 22
Brown, J., 3, 5, 6, 42, 44
Brown, W., 95, 33
Brown, W. F., 48
Brutten, G. J., 167, 169, 172
Buckingham, H. W., 70

Subject Index

Page numbers in italics refer to illustrations; (T) refers to a table.

A

Ablation, of vocal tract structures, 10–12
Apraxia of speech, 5–8, 22–57
  assessment of, 42–50
  clinical neurophysiology in, 25
  diagnosis vs. assessment, 26–28
  neuroscience vs. phonetics approach to, 22–51
  treatment of, 42–50
  via nonspeech voluntary control tasks, 41
Articulation disorders, 3–57
  assessment of, 3–15
  from ablation of vocal tract structures, 10–12
  intervention strategies, 11–12
  neurologic, 5–10
  evaluation of, 5–9
  intervention strategies, 9–10
  treatment of, 3–15
Auditory stimulation, rhythmic, for treatment of stuttering, 159

B

Breathing, role of, in impaired vocal function, 91–92

C

Contrastive linguistics, 60

D

Disorders, of articulation. See *Articulation disorders.*
  of fluency. See *Fluency disorders.*
  phonologic. See *Phonologic disorders.*
  vocal, 79–151 (see also *Voice disorders*)

D (cont.)

Dysarthria, 5–8, 22–57
  assessment of, 42–50
  clinical neurophysiology in, 25
  diagnosis vs. assessment, 26–28
  neuroscience vs. phonetics approach to, 22–51
  treatment of, 42–50
Dysphonia, spastic, 87–88, 99–100

E

Equivalence, in motor control of speech, *31*, 33–34

F

Filtering, inverse, for detection of laryngeal pathology, 82–83
Fluency, treated, normalcy of, 179–180, 196–198
Fluency disorders, emotional considerations of, 194–195, 197–198
  theories of, 155–158
  neurophysiologic, 157
  therapy for, 155–219
  altered speech patterns as a, 172–176
  anxiety reduction as a, 159–160
  attitudinal, 160–165, 198
  behavioral, 168
  clinical viability of, 199
  combination of various forms of, 176–177
  effect identification of, 189, 207–212
  evaluation of, 189–219
  follow-up evaluation after, 216–217, 193–194
  generalization of effects of, 150–182, 193
  maintenance of effects of, 180–182, 193–195, 199, 213–215

Phone substitution in native and taught
language, 63
Phonologic disorders, remediation of,
73-75
Phonologic processes of languages, 64-66
neutralization, 65
Phonologic systems, interaction of, 60-75
Phonosurgery, 97-100
Phonotactic differences of languages, 63
Pitch, perturbation of, as evidence of
vocal pathology, 83
Prosthetics, use of, in speech
rehabilitation, 114-115
Punishment, as a therapy for stuttering,
168-171

R

Reinterpretation of distinctions as a
phonologic interaction, 62
Respiration, role of, in voice disorders,
91-92

S

Second language, acquisition of, 59-75
pedagogic implications in, 70-73
stages in, 68(T)
variants in, 66-70
Spastic dysphonia. See *Dysphonia,
spastic.*
Spectral analysis of voice, 84
Speech, after stuttering treatment, clinical
vs. extraclinical performance
of, 193, 204-206
improvement of, as a result of
therapy, 195-196, 207
naturalness of, 196-197
normalcy of, 196-197, 200
apraxia of. See *Apraxia of speech.*
motor control process of, 21-24, 28-35
approaches used to evaluate, 44-50
components of, 23-25
equivalence in *31*, 33-34
hierachical form of, 30-32
vs. nonspeech activities, 35-42
Speech production, biologic process of,
24(T)
Speech quality measurement, for
stuttering therapy
evaluation, 203-204

Speech rate, for stuttering therapy
evaluation, 202-203
Speech rehabilitation, following
laryngectomy, 113-126
role of speech pathologists in, 24-25
surgical prosthetic approach to,
114-115
tracheoesophageal puncture approach
to, 115-117
prothesis used in, 122-124
nonspeech outcomes, 117-119
speech outcomes, 115-117
Stuttering, 155-219 (see also *Fluency
disorders*)
emotional considerations of, 194-195,
197-198
Stuttering frequency counts, for therapy
evaluation, 201-202
Substitution, of phones, in native and
taught language, 63

T

Therapy, for fluency disorders. See
*Fluency disorders, therapy
for.*
Tracheoesophageal puncture, patient
selection for, 120
Treated fluency, normalcy of, 179-180,
196-198

U

Ultrasound, as measure of laryngeal
impairment, 85
Underdifferentiation of contrastive
sounds, 61

V

VARP. See *Vocal Abuse Reduction
Program.*
Van Riper's therapy, 165-166
Video nasopharyngoscopy, as measure of
laryngeal impairment, 85
Vocal Abuse Reduction Program,
133-135, 138, 145